MW01108439

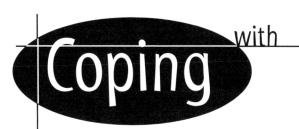

Coping with

CHEMOTHERAPY

Sandra Giddens and Owen Giddens

The Rosen Publishing Group, Inc.
New York

Dedicated to our children, Justine and Kyle, with love

Published in 2001 by The Rosen Publishing Group, Inc.
29 East 21st Street, New York, NY 10010

Cover photo © David Turnley/Corbis

Library of Congress Cataloging-in-Publication Data

Giddens, Sandra.
Coping with chemotherapy / by Sandra and Owen
Giddens.— 1st ed.
p. cm. — (Coping)
ISBN 0-8239-3361-X
1. Cancer—Chemotherapy—Juvenile literature.
[1. Cancer—Chemotherapy. 2. Chemotherapy.]
I. Giddens, Owen. II. Title. III. Series.
RC271.C5 G53 2001
616.99'4061—dc21

2001000014

Manufactured in the United States of America

Contents

Introduction

The human spirit is stronger than anything that happens to it.
—C.C. Scott

Samuel and his family looked up at the doctor with anticipation, ready to find out the next course of action in their struggle to combat his cancer. It seemed as if the doctor paused for a long time before responding. Was there an answer? In the moment before the doctor spoke, the teenager and his family searched the doctor's eyes for some element of hope. Finally, the doctor looked up and said one word, "Chemotherapy." After much talk and clarification, they all decided that this was in fact the best way to deal with the cancer. Looking back on that day, Samuel realized that his struggle was only just beginning.

Learning that you may have to undergo chemotherapy can trigger many emotions. You are learning not only to deal with having cancer but also how to eradicate it from your system. Up to this point, your focus may have always been on instant gratification, having a great time with your

1

friends, going out on weekends, and talking about what's happening at school. When you find out you have cancer, your health becomes your focus. Coping with chemotherapy entails keeping yourself strong so you can fight the cancer cells in your body. Chemotherapy is hard on your body; there is no denying that fact. There are side effects that range from mild to severe, and many side effects are unpleasant—both emotionally and physically. Sometimes you will feel in control, and at other times you will want someone to assist you.

Ideally, when you undergo chemotherapy treatments you put yourself in the hands of competent and knowledgeable people who are there to help you. The oncologists (doctors who specialize in cancer), nurses, social workers, psychologists, hospital volunteers, and X-ray technicians have one ultimate goal: to help you live longer and hopefully cancer free.

This can be a vulnerable time. You not only have to deal with physical difficulties, such as recovering from surgery, but also emotional issues. You may wonder, "Will I survive?" You will need support from people around you, and, most important, you will need to draw on your own personal strength to help fight this disease.

It can be a mind-boggling experience to be told you have cancer. It is also traumatic to hear that one method of treatment involves pumping the body with drugs—many of them poisonous and with harsh side effects. Is the gamble worth it? Are the pain and suffering worth it? Is it the answer to your prayers? Many children, teens, and adults who have gone through chemotherapy answer yes. Even though chemotherapy can be physically and emotionally draining, most survivors said they would go through it again. Why? Because they are alive and here to tell their stories.

The August 7, 2000, issue of *The Globe and Mail*, a Toronto daily newspaper, featured an article about the athlete Lance Armstrong, who fought cancer with chemotherapy treatments. The following is an excerpt from that article.

> *Cycling icon Lance Armstrong was slipping back in the pack: The cocky, brash Texan, normally so full of steam, had wilted in the 220 kilometer road race during the 1996 Summer Games in Atlanta . . . What no one realized, least of all the athlete himself, was that cancer was galloping through his body. The surprise wasn't that he finished twelfth in the race, it was that he finished at all. A diagnosis of late-stage testicular cancer at the age of twenty-five threatened to put him out of the game for good . . . Armstrong faced a forty percent chance of survival. If this was the early 1970s, he would have surely died . . . Armstrong's chemotherapy treatments started. He rolled himself into a fetal position, retching around the clock. "On the really bad days, I would lie on my side in bed, wrapped in blankets, fighting the noxious roiling in my stomach and the fever raging under my skin," [said Armstrong.] "I'd peek out from under the blankets and just grunt." Despite the weakness and loss of hair, including even his eyelashes, there were days he would cycle fifty to eighty kilometers. "Chemo had made the worst climb in the Alps seem flat,"* he wrote in his autobiography, It's Not About the Bike: My Journey Back to Life. *And yet the same Lance Armstrong*

learned he will lead the five-man U.S. road team to race for gold at the Sydney Olympics in 2000. If that wasn't enough, two weeks ago he also won the Tour de France.

In the following chapters, you will read the true stories of children, teens, and adults who, like Armstrong, have all gone through chemotherapy. You will hear their personal accounts as well as the memories of their family members. You will also meet oncologists and learn how they work with cancer patients.

Cancer

The longer I live, the more beautiful life becomes.
                                        —Frank Lloyd Wright

Our bodies are made up of millions and millions of cells. Cells are so tiny that they can be seen only through a microscope. In the center of each cell is a nucleus, the cell's command center. Within the nucleus, there are thousands and thousands of genes that determine everything about that individual cell. To replace worn-out cells, certain genes direct the cell to divide into two exact copies. When there is a mutation, or change, in the genes, these cells continue to divide, even when the cell does not need to replace itself. The mutation can cause the new cell to be different from the original cell. We still do not fully understand what causes these cells to mutate.

These cells have now become so different that they are abnormal and continue to grow and divide and grow and divide, again and again. These uncontrolled cells are cancer cells. Cancer cells often ignore the normal rate of cell division because they lack a growth-control mechanism. Normal cells have a tendency to remain together in their individual body organs, but cancer cells are more likely to detach themselves from their original location and move by way of the bloodstream to other organs in the body.

Tumors

As more and more of these cancerous cells form, they come together into a mass called a tumor. This tumor, which is made up of cancer cells, is said to be malignant (nocuous). One tumor the size of a pea could contain as many as a billion cancer cells. Tumors can grow to any shape or size. They can even become as big as a melon. Nonsolid tumors consist of cancer cells that develop in fluids (like blood) or tissue and travel throughout the body.

Normal cells can also grow into a tumor, but they do not contain cancer cells. These are benign (innocuous) tumors. A pathology report can usually determine whether a tumor is benign or malignant.

Causes of Cancer

Cancer is a generic term for a couple of hundred similar but distinct diseases that advance and spread at different rates. Imagine that your body is a well-tuned machine. Your cells, tissues, and organs are busy working all the time in your body. They work day and night to keep you alive. Anything that interferes with their functioning disrupts the operation of your well-tuned machine. Vital organs like your brain, liver, kidneys, and blood require smooth maintenance at all times. Cancer can disrupt this whole cycle and jeopardize the ability of your body to function properly.

No one knows for sure how a normal cell becomes a cancer cell. We do know of several things that cause cancer. When nuclear bombs were dropped in 1945 at the end of World War II on the Japanese cities of Nagasaki and Hiroshima, people were exposed to radiation poisoning. Many, many people developed cancer from this radiation. We also know that firsthand and secondhand smoking of tobacco causes cancer. Nearly six out of seven people with lung cancer have smoked. Benzene, which is a liquid from coal tar used to make dyes, can cause cancer. Exposure to asbestos, which was once used in building construction, can also lead to cancer. Excessive exposure to the ultraviolet rays of the sun can cause skin cancer.

Warning Signs

Cancer can strike people at any age, from very young to very old. It is more likely to occur in older people. Approximately 1 out of 3 adults will have cancer. Approximately 1 out of every 10,000 children will develop cancer. Here are some warning signs that may indicate that cancer cells are present in the body. These signs do not necessarily mean you have cancer, but they should be checked out by your family physician.

☞ Changes in a mole

☞ Changes in a wart

⮑ Sores that do not heal

⮑ New or unusual body lumps

⮑ Persistent coughing or hoarseness

⮑ Chronic pain

⮑ Chronic fever

⮑ Unusual bleeding, such as blood in the urine or in the stool

⮑ Unexplained weakness, weight loss, or fatigue

It is difficult to detect some forms of cancer. Some people in the early stages of cancer do not recover, and others in advanced stages are cured. We do know some important protective measures.

⮑ Don't smoke.

⮑ If you smoke, quit.

⮑ Avoid secondhand smoke.

⮑ Protect your skin with strong sunscreen.

⮑ Avoid exposure to carcinogens like radiation and asbestos.

⮑ Eat healthful foods.

⮑ Have regular medical checkups.

☞ If you have a strong family history of cancer, especially of breast or uterine cancer, seek genetic counseling.

☞ If you have a strong family history of colon cancer, talk to your doctor.

Diagnosis

As there are many types of cancer, there are a number of different tests to confirm a cancer diagnosis. For instance, if you found a lump in your breast, you would go to the doctor. The doctor would then order a mammogram. A mammogram is an X ray of the breast. If the mammogram revealed a suspicious mass, the doctor would have to investigate further to determine if the lump was benign or malignant. The doctor might try to withdraw fluid from the lump with a needle. Clear fluid would probably mean the lump was harmless. If no fluid came out, the most likely next step would be for you to go to the hospital for a biopsy (surgical removal of tissue from the lump). The doctor would send this tissue to the laboratory, where technicians would perform tests to determine if the lump was cancerous.

Doctors also use computed tomography (CT) or computed axial tomography (CAT) scans to look inside your body. This CT or CAT scan provides doctors with a detailed cross-sectional view of the inside of your body. The CAT scan enables the doctor to see tumors and identify types of tumors. If cancer is present, the CAT scan shows where it is in the body.

Types of Cancer

The most common cancers start in the:

⇌ Lungs

⇌ Colon or rectum

⇌ Blood

⇌ Ovaries

⇌ Breasts

⇌ Pancreas

⇌ Prostate

⇌ Skin

Cancer that starts from a lung cell is called lung cancer. But if breast cancer cells spread to a lung and form tumors, doctors continue to refer to those new secondary tumors as breast cancer, not lung cancer. Can you think of an organ where cancer cannot grow? The heart is the only one. Heart cells do not divide or replace themselves.

Stages of the Disease

Doctors assess the condition of their cancer patients according to stages. They determine the stage according to the following:

⇌ Size of the tumor

⇌ Location of the cancer cells

☞ Amount of healthy tissue affected

☞ Rapidity with which the cancer is spreading

The more advanced the cancer, the higher the stage. Stage one cancer is relatively mild; stage four is far more severe. For example, a patient with a small tumor that has not metastasized, or spread, has a stage one condition. If the cancer has already spread to vital organs and secondary tumors are growing, doctors categorize the cancer as stage four. Of course, stage four cancer is far more difficult to cure. When your body is infested with cancer cells, these cells must be destroyed. One way to destroy these cells is chemotherapy.

Chemotherapy

Chemotherapy research dates back to World War II. A ship full of American soldiers was carrying a deadly mustard gas. There was an explosion on the ship that killed many soldiers. Pathologists, who study the nature of diseases, examined some of the dead bodies. The damage the gas caused to the lymph system and bone marrow amazed these pathologists.

After the war, physicians at Yale University started to experiment with gases. They worked with a related gas, called nitrogen mustard, to see how it might affect cancers of the blood and lymph system. Their initial investigations revealed that the treatment temporarily reduced the size of tumors. This was the beginning of chemotherapy. Over the years, researchers in government-sponsored programs have tested more than a quarter of a million drugs that they have hoped would combat cancer.

How Chemotherapy Works

Once cancer is diagnosed, the next step is treatment. Chemotherapy is the use of drugs to treat cancer. These drugs are often called anticancer drugs. Chemotherapy drugs disrupt the cancer cells' ability to grow and multiply.

These medications destroy cancer cells without permanently damaging the normal cells in the body. One important thing about cancer cells, unlike normal cells, is that they are not able to repair themselves once damaged.

Doctors use chemotherapy to eradicate small, nearly invisible tumors, or to shrink larger tumors prior to surgery (if surgery is necessary). Chemotherapy may also be used after surgery to eliminate remaining cancer cells that have spread to other parts of the body. Many doctors choose chemotherapy for their cancer patients because it destroys these small, nearly invisible cancer cells that exist in the body.

Chemotherapy consists of one or more drugs that act in different ways to destroy cancer cells. The type of chemotherapy a doctor administers to a patient depends on the type of cancer he or she suffers from, where it is located in the body, and the stage of its growth. Depending on the type of cancer and its stage of development, chemotherapy can be used to:

➷ Cure cancer

➷ Slow the cancer's growth

➷ Prevent cancer from spreading

➷ Relieve symptoms

Different chemotherapy drugs work in different ways. Some chemotherapy drugs affect cancer cells during the process of cell division. If a cell cannot divide, it will eventually die. Other drugs make the environment less hospitable for the cancer cell. Doctors try to destroy most cancer cells during the first round of chemotherapy. Then they allow the body time to recover before administering another cycle of chemotherapy and hopefully eliminating the remaining cancer cells.

Designing a Treatment Plan

A doctor designs an individual treatment plan, or protocol, for each patient. A protocol is a road map or a plan of action. Protocols provide guidelines for:

↪ What treatments should be used

↪ Appropriate doses of drugs

↪ Treatment schedules

↪ What diagnostic tests should be done to evaluate how one is responding to the treatment

↪ What changes must be made if the cancer cells are not responding as expected

Each protocol is tailor-made for and specific to each patient. How often and how long you receive chemotherapy depends on the kind of cancer you have, the goals of treatment, the drugs that are used, and how your body responds to the treatments. A person may need to receive chemotherapy every day, every week, or every month. It is often given in cycles, so that your body has some time to rest and recuperate. These rest periods also give normal cells a chance to grow.

Administering Chemotherapy

Depending on the type of chemotherapy your doctor chooses, you could receive your drugs as an inpatient in a hospital, by visiting a clinic, or at home. Chemotherapy can be administered in the following ways.

Intravenously (IV): There are different intravenous methods. In most cases, chemotherapy drugs are injected into a vein. The doctor may decide to put the line in your arm. This is called a peripherally inserted central-venous catheter, or a PICC line.

When an IV is inserted, it feels like having blood drawn for a blood test. Many people experience a sensation of coolness. Some people have little or no difficulty having the IV in their hand or their lower arm.

Chemotherapy drugs can be diluted into a large bag of liquid and administered by a "drip" into a vein. The drugs are then inserted into the vein through a thin needle, usually in the hand or lower arm. A fine tube, or cannula, is inserted into the vein and taped securely to the arm.

Another intravenous method involves the insertion of a plastic tube or central line into a vein in the chest. Once the central line is in place, it is either stitched or taped to the chest to prevent it from being pulled out of the vein. It can remain in the vein for many months. There are two potential risks associated with this method: infection and blockage. To prevent these complications, once or twice a week the line has to be flushed with the preventive drug heparin.

Yet another intravenous method uses a catheter, also known as a Hickman line. The catheter is a thin tube inserted in a large vein in the heart. A doctor installs the tube during a very brief operation. The Hickman line enables doctors to administer drugs rapidly. The portacap is a variation on the Hickman line. It is a port, or a small plastic or metal container, implanted under the skin connected to a tube inserted in a vein.

Sometimes it is difficult to insert the needle into the vein, and the doctor may decide that a central-venous catheter or port is the preferred method of treatment. Both these treatments avoid the insertion of the needle into the vein or even damaging the veins. Central-venous catheters and ports do not cause pain or discomfort if they are properly placed and, of course, monitored. Any pain associated with the aforementioned procedures should be reported to a nurse or doctor immediately.

Orally: Chemotherapy can be administered in pill, capsule, or liquid form. Capsules or tablets can be taken at home. Doctors determine the dosage and inform patients of special restrictions and side effects associated with these drugs.

Intermuscularly: Doctors inject the drugs under the skin or directly into the cancerous area.

Intrathecally: Used in very special cases, this method entails injecting chemotherapy drugs into the fluid around the spine.

Topically: Chemotherapy can be applied directly to the skin.

By Infusion Pump: Infusion pumps are portable pumps, and they release a controlled amount of chemotherapy drugs into the bloodstream over a period of time. The pumps are quite small and portable; most are battery operated.

Regardless of method, as soon as the chemotherapy drugs are administered, they are absorbed into the bloodstream and carried throughout the body, hopefully reaching all of the cancerous cells.

Monitoring

Doctors rely on regular blood tests, physical examinations, and other diagnostic tools to monitor how the body responds to chemotherapy treatments. Constant monitoring is necessary to find out how cancer cells are responding to treatment. Doctors also need to monitor damage chemotherapy drugs might inflict on the body's healthy organs. Some drugs affect particular organs such as the heart, liver, and kidneys. Through monitoring, doctors make sure that the body has recovered from the previous cycle of chemotherapy.

Chemotherapy may be administered before or after surgery. It may be administered on its own or in combination with radiation therapy. Radiation therapy is the use of radiation to shrink and damage cancer cells in a specific area of the body. Radiation destroys cells by eliminating their ability to reproduce.

Unfortunately, chemotherapy drugs seek out and destroy not only cancer cells but also normal cells that are rapidly dividing. The normal cells most likely to be affected are those located in the gastrointestinal tract, hair, and bone marrow. Unlike cancer cells, the great thing about one's normal cells is their ability to recover quickly once chemotherapy stops.

Questions for Your Oncologist

↝ How will chemotherapy treat my type of cancer?

↝ Explain my protocol. What drugs make up the protocol and what are their side effects?

↝ Where will my chemotherapy be performed? In the hospital or as an outpatient?

↝ If I am hospitalized, how long do you think I will be there?

↝ Are any preparations necessary beforehand, like blood tests?

↝ Will I have to be operated on?

↪ Will I be sedated? If so, what drug or drugs will I be given and how? Intravenously? Orally?

↪ Are there any health risks associated with the chemotherapy drugs? If so, explain them to me.

↪ Can I expect any pain?

↪ What is the actual procedure like?

↪ How long will each session take and how many sessions will I undergo?

↪ When will the results be available, and who will inform me of them?

↪ How will the chemotherapy be administered?

↪ How long until my hair falls out. Will it fall out all over my body?

↪ Are there any drugs you recommend for nausea?

↪ What should I do if I develop sores in my mouth?

↪ Will you give me the same protocol each time or change it?

↪ What side effects should I expect and how will you relieve them?

↪ Are the side effects temporary or permanent?

⇒ Do I have to be on a special diet?

⇒ Will I experience infertility?

⇒ What is the latest research on my type of cancer?

⇒ Are there any side effects that I should report immediately?

⇒ Are there any alternative treatment methods I could consider?

Other Medication

Some medications can interfere with the effects of your chemotherapy. Before beginning your treatments, take all medications to your doctor to discuss their effects on the anticancer drugs. You should make a list of over-the-counter drugs like laxatives, cold pills, pain relievers, and vitamins you use regularly. Your doctor will also want to know how often you take medication, the dose, and the reason. The doctor will discuss which drugs will not affect your chemotherapy and which ones you should avoid. Also, ask your doctor if drinking alcohol will affect your chemotherapy.

Paying for Chemotherapy

In Canada, the national health system insures chemotherapy treatments, freeing patients from payment concerns. Most health insurance policies in the United States cover at least part if not all of the costs of many kinds of chemotherapy. The cost in the States can vary according to the drug protocol and overall treatment plan. In some states, Medicaid may help pay for certain treatments. If you need help financing your chemotherapy, contact your hospital's social service office, the Cancer Information Service, the American Cancer Society, or your state or county social service agency.

Physical Side Effects

Each patient responds differently to his or her drug regimen or protocol. As the parent of one patient explained, "To fight a headache, you may need one aspirin, another person may need two, and another may need to take something even stronger. Each person is unique and reacts to chemotherapy in his or her own manner." The following is an extensive outline of some of the side effects of chemotherapy. Keep in mind that you may not necessarily experience them all.

Hair Loss

All the patients interviewed for this book knew that chemotherapy often causes hair loss. For some, hair loss was devastating; others took it in stride. Some wore wigs; some were comfortable being seen bald. Hair loss can occur on all parts of your body. It is not restricted just to your head. Hair on your face, legs, underarms, and pubic area can all be affected.

Hair can fall out gradually or in big clumps after chemotherapy treatments. Hair usually grows back a

couple of months after the completion of the chemotherapy treatments. The hair that does grow back may have a
different texture or color. It may be dull and dry in
appearance. Here are some suggestions as to how to care
for your hair before and during chemotherapy treatments.

⮩ Use mild shampoos.

⮩ Use a brush with soft hair bristles.

⮩ Avoid permanent waves or dyeing your hair.

⮩ Use the low heat on your blow-dryer.

⮩ Do not use brush rollers or heated rollers.

⮩ To protect your scalp from the sun, remember sunscreen
and wear a hat or a scarf.

⮩ Get fitted for a wig before your treatments.

Wigs

A good synthetic wig can cost up to $350. But you can
also purchase used wigs. In fact, the American Cancer
Society has wig banks. Your nurse or social worker can put
you in touch with a wig bank. The following are tips on
wearing and maintaining a wig.

⮩ Brush your remaining hair.

⮩ Try to have your wig fitted privately. If you have
already lost your hair, questions posed to you by
others may be insensitive.

⮕ After your wig has been fitted, have it styled.

⮕ Make sure your wig is placed on your head properly. Your hairline should start four finger widths from the top of your eyebrows.

⮕ Wash your wig approximately once every three weeks in cold water with special wig shampoo.

⮕ Do not brush or comb the wig when it is wet.

⮕ A little mousse can be used to shape the wig.

⮕ When chemotherapy is completed, donate your wig to a wig bank to help other patients.

Gastrointestinal Symptoms

When you start your treatments, you might experience nausea, vomiting, diarrhea, constipation, and/or loss of appetite. There are medications that relieve nausea and vomiting. These gastrointestinal (GI) symptoms usually disappear after you have completed the chemotherapy treatments.

Nausea and Vomiting

Patients may experience nausea and vomiting depending on the chemotherapy drugs administered and how their bodies respond to the drugs. Many people feel nauseous and vomit. Some people do not experience these side effects at all. Some people feel nauseous for short periods of time while others feel nauseous and vomit daily.

24

It is important to report your symptoms to your nurse or doctor so that he or she can remedy the nausea and/or vomiting. Also, to ensure that you do not become dehydrated from too much vomiting, seek medical advice immediately. Your doctor may prescribe antiemetics, which are drugs that curb these symptoms. If an anti-nausea drug is not working, ask to receive another. The following are further suggestions as to how to cope with nausea and vomiting.

- Eat small meals throughout the day.

- Drink liquids at least an hour before or after your meal, instead of with your meal.

- Avoid strong odors like tobacco smoke, perfume, and strong spices.

- Stay away from sweet, fried, or fatty foods.

- Suck on ice cubes or mints.

- Eat and drink slowly.

- Chew your food well for easier digestion.

- Avoid eating for at least a few hours before treatment if nausea occurs during or right after treatment.

- If morning nausea persists, try eating foods like cereal, crackers, or toast. (If you have mouth or throat sores, or if you are having difficulty wetting your mouth with saliva, do not eat these foods.)

∽ Drink cool, clear, unsweetened fruit juices such as apple and grape juice, or flat ginger ale.

∽ Rest in a chair after eating, but do not lie prone for at least two hours after you have finished eating.

∽ Breathe deeply and slowly when you feel nauseous.

∽ Try meditation.

∽ Use relaxation techniques.

∽ Do not wear tight-fitting clothes.

∽ Listen to calming music.

∽ Distract yourself by chatting with friends or family members, listening to music, watching television or a video, etc.

Diarrhea

When you have diarrhea, food moves through your large intestines so quickly that your body does not absorb water properly. Consequently, your bowel movements are more liquid and more frequent. Repeated episodes of diarrhea can be both a physical and an emotional strain. They can cause severe fluid loss and imbalances in the salts and minerals your body requires; they can also be embarrassing.

How does chemotherapy cause diarrhea? Chemotherapy and radiation therapy can damage the cells in the intestinal tract that are dividing frequently. The body responds by trying to remove the damaged tissue as quickly as possible.

Anything in the intestines moves out in the form of liquid stools or diarrhea. This clears up when the intestinal tract heals. Diarrhea can also be caused by the medications given to prevent nausea or by an infection. If you are experiencing diarrhea:

- Drink lots of fluids.

- Sip fruit juices, nectars, soups, or sport drinks that replace your electrolytes.

- Drink moderately cool or lukewarm liquids.

- Take the fizz out of sodas like ginger ale.

- Keep an accurate record of your weight.

Constipation

Some people become constipated after ingesting chemotherapy drugs and/or the painkilling drugs they receive. Others may become constipated because they are less active and eating less than usual. Emotional stress can also contribute to changes in bowel movements.

Tell your doctor if you have not had a bowel movement for more than a couple of days. You may need to use a stool softener or a laxative. Do not use anything until you have checked with your doctor or nurse, especially if your white blood cell count is low. Enemas or suppositories may cause infection if your white blood cell level is low. If your white blood cell count is low, you should also avoid raw fruits and vegetables, including lettuce. These foods normally function as dietary remedies for constipation. A few ways to help prevent constipation:

➯ Exercise regularly.

➯ Eat a high-fiber diet that includes whole grains, fruits, vegetables, dried fruits, and fruit juices (unless blood counts are low or your doctor does not recommend it).

➯ Drink lots of fluids.

➯ Avoid refined foods like candy and white bread.

➯ Avoid foods like chocolate, cheese, and eggs, which can cause constipation.

Changes in Blood Cell Count

Fatigue and Anemia

Many patients complain of exhaustion after chemotherapy treatments. Exhaustion may also be due in part to anemia. A low number of red blood cells can put a cancer patient into an anemic state. More than 50 percent of people, young and old, undergoing chemotherapy experience anemia. The possible side effects of anemia are fatigue, paleness, and lightheadedness. This is because normal tissues in the body are not receiving enough oxygen.

Doctors constantly monitor blood cell count during chemotherapy. If your red blood cell count falls too low, you may need a blood transfusion. The transfusion will increase the number of red blood cells in your body. Here are some things that may also help alleviate anemia.

- ➣ Eat a well-balanced diet.

- ➣ Eat foods rich in iron, such as liver, red meat, or leafy green vegetables.

- ➣ Before going to bed, avoid foods containing caffeine, such as coffee, chocolate, or colas.

- ➣ Drink a lot of water and other liquids.

- ➣ Rise slowly from sitting or lying down to prevent dizziness.

- ➣ Get plenty of rest. If you can, take naps during the day.

- ➣ Limit strenuous activities.

- ➣ If you know you have a social event in the evening, rest during the day to conserve your energy.

Infection

Chemotherapy also affects white blood cells. These are the cells that fight infection. As with your red cell count, your white blood cell count will be checked regularly. If your white blood cell count does drop, your doctor may postpone your next chemotherapy treatment or give you a lower dose of drugs. It is important to try to prevent infections by taking the following precautionary measures.

29

➥ Clean cuts and scrapes right away with warm water, soap, and an antiseptic.

➥ Try to avoid contact with people who have a contagious illness.

➥ Try to avoid contact with children who have recently received immunizations, such as vaccines for polio, measles, mumps, and rubella (German measles).

➥ Try to stay away from crowds.

➥ Avoid raw eggs, raw milk, and stagnant water.

➥ Take a warm bath or shower every day.

➥ Wash your hands often.

➥ Clean your rectal area thoroughly after each bowel movement.

Warning Signs

Stay alert to the following signs which may indicate infection.

➥ Fever over 100 degrees Fahrenheit or 37.5 degrees Celsius

➥ Sweating

➥ Chills

➥ A burning sensation when you urinate

➥ A severe cough

⮞ A severe sore throat

⮞ Severe diarrhea

⮞ Redness or swelling, especially around wounds, sores, pimples, or intravenous catheter sites

It is vital that you report any signs of infection to your doctor immediately. Do not wait. This is especially a concern if your white blood cell count is low. If you have a fever, do not use aspirin, acetaminophen, or any other medicine to reduce your temperature without first consulting your doctor.

If you are going on vacation, it is important not to have any "live virus" vaccines. These vaccines include polio, measles, rubella (German measles), MMM (the triple vaccine for measles, mumps, and rubella), BCG (tuberculosis), yellow fever, and oral typhoid. Ask your doctor which vaccines are safe for you. Other vaccines—such as those for diphtheria, tetanus, flu, hepatitis A, hepatitis B, rabies, cholera, and typhoid—should all be approved by your doctor as well.

Mouth and Throat Discomfort

Some patients complain of mucositis or stomatitis. Mucositis is an inflammation of the mucous membranes in the gastrointestinal system. These mucous membranes line the mouth, throat, esophagus, and the rest of the digestive tract. Many patients also complain of sores in the mouth.

31

Stomatitis refers specifically to an inflammation of the mucous membranes in your mouth. If sores develop in your esophagus, you have developed esophagitis.

During the months you receive chemotherapy treatments, there may be times when your mouth and throat become sore. Initially, patients may experience a hypersensitivity to sour or spicy tastes. They may also notice some redness or swelling in the gums, cheeks, mouth palate, or throat. They may eventually develop open sores similar to cold sores. Seemingly routine and simple activities—like brushing the teeth, eating, or swallowing—may become painful.

These problems occur when the surface layer of cells that line your mouth or your throat is not replaced quickly enough because of your treatments. While you are experiencing these mouth sores, here are some things you can do to promote healing and prevent infection.

- See a dentist to have your teeth cleaned before you start chemotherapy.

- Take care of any cavities, abscesses, gum disease, etc.

- Chemotherapy can make you more susceptible to cavities. Your dentist may suggest using a fluoride rinse or gel each day to help prevent decay.

- Rinse your mouth within thirty minutes after meals.

- Use a toothbrush with soft bristles. (Wet bristles with hot water to soften them; let cool before brushing.)

32

↬ Use a sponge-tipped swab if brushing is too difficult.

↬ Use a mouth rinse. You can use one half-teaspoon of baking soda mixed with one half-cup of water (125 ml.). Commercial mouthwashes containing alcohol or glycerine are not recommended at this time, as they may dry your mouth.

↬ If mouth dryness bothers you, ask your doctor if you should use an artificial saliva product to moisten your mouth.

↬ Avoid hot and spicy foods.

↬ Avoid hot drinks.

↬ Avoid acidic drinks like orange and grapefruit juices that may sting.

↬ For severe mouth pain, rinse with a topical anesthetic.

↬ Avoid irritating acidic foods such as tomatoes and citrus fruit. Avoid rough, coarse, or dry foods such as raw vegetables, granola, and toast.

↬ A diet containing adequate vitamins, minerals, and protein can speed the healing of the mucous membranes.

↬ Consult a nutritionist to ensure that you maintain a well-balanced diet.

Dryness of Skin and Nails

A number of factors, including chemotherapy, antinausea medication, dehydration, or poor nutrition, cause dry skin. Radiation therapy can affect skin as well. Chemotherapy also makes your skin more sensitive to the sun's rays. This means you may burn easily. Some chemotherapy drugs also cause darkening of the skin under the nails, over joints, or of the mucous membranes in your mouth.

If you receive chemotherapy through the veins of your hands or your arms, you may develop a darkening of the skin over the veins. You may look at your arms and see the patterns of your veins outlined in a color several shades darker than your normal skin tone.

Chemotherapy can also cause your nails to become brittle and grow at a slower rate than usual. Your nails may also become very soft. As a result, they are more likely to rip. Here are some ways you can care for your skin and nails.

⇒ Lubricate your skin with moisturizers and oils.

⇒ Take warm baths or showers; hot water can dry skin.

⇒ Use a moisturizing soap.

⇒ Avoid scratchy materials like wool next to your skin.

⇒ Avoid alcohol-based products.

⇒ Use sunscreen with a high protection level.

⇒ Use lip-gloss with sunscreen to protect your lips.

⇒ Wear long-sleeved shirts and long pants for protection from the sun.

☞ Trim or clip your nails regularly.

☞ Do not use artificial nails at this time.

☞ Use a lanolin-based rather than an alcohol-based polish or polish remover.

Sexual Activity

Many people go through chemotherapy treatments and their sex lives remain unaffected. You may lose interest in sex because you are exhausted from the treatments. The stress of the treatments and the anxiety of having cancer can weigh heavily on your mind.

However, there is no medical reason to stop having sex during chemotherapy as long as you use adequate protection. If you are concerned that chemotherapy will affect your sex life, talk with your doctor or nurse. If you have a sexual partner, this is also the time to communicate with each other, sharing your worries and concerns.

Fertility

Oncologists always explain the risk of infertility to their patients. Although fertility may not be at the forefront of a young patient's mind, such concerns are addressed, as some chemotherapy drugs do cause infertility. Whether you are male or female, learning that your chemotherapy treatments might cause infertility can be upsetting.

The treatments can cause temporary infertility and premature menopause in women. Also, monthly periods may become irregular or eventually stop altogether. Men can become sterile from or temporarily impotent during chemotherapy treatments. Infertility may be temporary or permanent depending on which drugs you receive. It is very important that you discuss fertility concerns with your doctor before starting chemotherapy treatments.

For Women: Most drugs do not affect your fertility, but some drugs may affect your ovaries. The ovaries may stop producing eggs. If this does occur, you can no longer become pregnant, and you will probably experience symptoms of menopause. You may also experience hot flashes, dry skin, and dryness of the vagina. To help prevent these side effects, your doctor may prescribe hormone treatments or suggest a cream or ointment that helps moisten the vagina.

If infertility is short-lived, after your chemotherapy treatments finish, your periods will return to normal. About one-third of women experience infertility on a short-term basis. The younger you are, the more likely it is that normal periods will return and that you will still be able to have children when treatments cease.

Women should try to avoid becoming pregnant during chemotherapy treatments, as the drugs may affect the fetus. Your doctor will talk to you about appropriate birth control methods. Usually condoms or other barrier methods of contraception are recommended. If you are pregnant before your chemotherapy starts, it is imperative that you consult your doctor. Postponing chemotherapy until the baby is born will be an option, but it will depend on the type of cancer you have, the extent of the cancer, and the drugs used in your protocol.

For Men: While some drugs may reduce the number of sperm you produce or affect the sperms' ability to reach and fertilize a woman's egg, it is very important that throughout your treatment you use a reliable form of contraception. You will be able to have an erection and orgasm as you did before treatment.

If you are concerned about infertility and want children in the near future, you may consider banking your sperm at a sperm bank for later use. Your sperm samples will be frozen and stored. Later, your partner could be impregnated artificially. Try to locate a bank close to where you live and inquire about the cost of this service.

Your doctor can perform a sperm count during and after your treatments. Infertility caused by chemotherapy is sometimes temporary, but in some cases it can be permanent. In other cases, fertility is restored a few years after the completion of chemotherapy treatments.

Other Physical Concerns

Some chemotherapy drugs produce side effects on the nervous system or the muscles. These side effects manifest themselves in tingling, numbness, weakness, or burning sensations in the hands and feet. You may also experience difficulties with your motor coordination and/or a loss of balance. Some people sense pain in the jaw and stomach. Some patients also suffer from hearing loss. If you experience any of these side effects, be sure to report them to your doctor immediately.

Some drugs can cause temporary or permanent damage to the kidneys or irritate the bladder. A few chemotherapy drugs cause urine to turn orange or red and may change the odor. Some drugs will cause semen to change color. Notify your doctor if you develop any of the following symptoms:

- ➥ Pain or burning when you urinate

- ➥ Frequent urination

- ➥ Reddish or bloody urine

- ➥ Fever

- ➥ Chills

- ➥ A sense that you need to urinate immediately

Some chemotherapy drugs cause your body to retain fluids. Your body, including your face, may appear puffy. On the scale you may be gaining weight, but this weight gain actually results from fluid retention. Talk to your doctor about this condition. Your doctor may prescribe diuretics (medicines that alleviate excess fluid buildup). Remember to avoid excess salt. In general, it is a good idea to keep a close eye on bodily changes throughout treatment.

The chemotherapy drugs that you are taking may have a number of potential side effects. You may be fortunate to experience few or no symptoms. You can look to pamphlets, booklets, books, and research tools like the Internet to educate yourself about the drugs doctors prescribe. Asking the nurse or the doctor to explain will also help you understand each drug and its side effects. It is also very important not to be embarrassed when you are experiencing a side effect. A doctor or nurse can suggest ways to relieve you of these symptoms. Remember, the more you share with your doctors and nurses, the more you will realize that you are not alone.

Emotional Responses

Undergoing chemotherapy introduces not only major physical changes but also a great deal of emotional stress into patients' lives. Chemotherapy affects their overall health, threatens their sense of well-being, disrupts their daily lives, and strains their personal relationships. Although people frequently talk about the physical side effects of chemotherapy, there are also emotional side effects. During this time, you will face extraordinary pressures and challenges. With all these changes, many patients feel anxious, angry, depressed, frightened, or emotionally exhausted.

Depression

The stress and the fear involved in living with cancer and cancer treatment can cause deep sadness and, perhaps, deep depression. Doctors can recommend psychologists, psychiatrists, support groups, and social workers who can help patients talk about and process their feelings. Doctors can prescribe antidepressants as well. Depression, anxiety, and sleep disturbances are all conditions that need to be addressed, especially as they manifest themselves physically.

For instance, people who are depressed and anxious may not be eating or sleeping well.

Finding Support

If you are undergoing chemotherapy, these emotions are perfectly understandable and common, but they may also be disturbing. It is important that you find someone to talk to. You might choose a doctor, a nurse, a parent, a sibling, another family member, a close friend, or you may require the assistance of counseling professionals.

News of your illness and your treatments also affects people in your life. Some people whom you considered close may withdraw from you. They may be afraid of saying the wrong thing, or they may be emotionally unable to give you support. You can tell people that there is no "correct" thing to say to you, that being there and offering comfort is what you need.

There are many kinds of counselors who can help you express, understand, and work through emotions related to your chemotherapy treatments and your cancer. Depending on your preferences, needs, and financial resources, you may want to talk to a psychologist, psychiatrist, social worker, school guidance counselor, or a member of the clergy, such as a priest, minister, or rabbi. Here are some other suggestions.

➷ Find a self-help group associated with your hospital.

➷ Let your parents in on how you are feeling.

➥ Talk to your friends about your fears and anxieties.

➥ Talk to a cancer survivor.

➥ Discuss antidepression or antianxiety medication with your doctor.

Support Groups

Support groups help people who are going through or have gone through cancer treatments. Many people find that they can share thoughts and feelings with group members that they do not feel comfortable expressing to anyone else. Trained therapists run these support groups. Sometimes your doctor can put you in touch with a person your age who has gone through chemotherapy. You might be able to contact him or her by telephone, e-mail, or in person. It is very important not to keep your emotions bottled up inside. You need someone to talk to and to be there for you when you are feeling vulnerable.

Personal Strategies

While you are receiving chemotherapy, it is important to maintain a sense of physical and emotional balance. There are several methods you might use.

Try to have a positive attitude. As you go through your chemotherapy treatments, there will be days when you are feeling down and blue, but try to remain optimistic.

Try to maintain your strength emotionally and physically. There will be times when you are not hungry. Try to eat nourishing meals.

Become knowledgeable. Understand as much as you can about your cancer and your chemotherapy treatments. Reading books on the subject, consulting Web sites and videos, and talking to people, as well as reviewing brochures and booklets from the hospital, can keep you informed.

Ask questions. It does not matter how silly you think your questions are. It is important that you feel satisfied that all your questions have been answered. Knowledge can help lessen some of the stress you may be feeling.

Keep a journal or diary. A record of your thoughts, feelings, or day-to-day events like the side effects you experience can help you through treatment. If you are unwell, ask a family member to keep the journal or diary until you are ready to take over. This process also creates a valuable personal history. It can be an amazing feeling to look back over the years and see how you survived. You might also gain great pleasure from knowing that your bout with cancer is in the past.

Set realistic goals for yourself. Many side effects of chemotherapy are very harsh. Do not be too hard on yourself. You probably will not have the energy that you once had while you undergo treatment. Remember, your body is fighting as hard as it can to remove cancerous cells.

Exercise a little if you can. By doing some exercise you can relieve some tension and anger as well as work up an appetite. Ask your doctor, nurse, or social worker about a suitable exercise program.

Take up a hobby. You could try knitting, needlepoint, joining a choir, or reading.

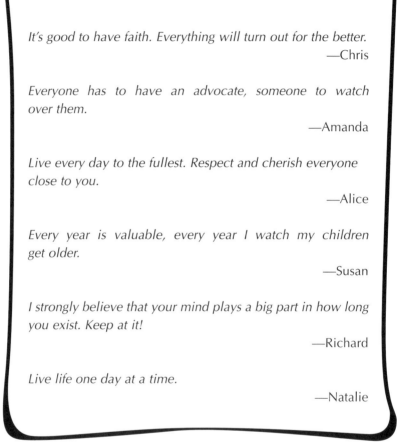

Encouraging Words from Cancer Survivors

It's good to have faith. Everything will turn out for the better.
—Chris

Everyone has to have an advocate, someone to watch over them.
—Amanda

Live every day to the fullest. Respect and cherish everyone close to you.
—Alice

Every year is valuable, every year I watch my children get older.
—Susan

I strongly believe that your mind plays a big part in how long you exist. Keep at it!
—Richard

Live life one day at a time.
—Natalie

Relieving Stress

If you undergo chemotherapy, it is important that you do everything in your power to keep your immune system strong. Relaxation techniques not only help you feel less overwhelmed but also reduce the immunity-suppressing

effects of stress. There are a variety of deep relaxation techniques. When you encounter particularly stressful days,
think about trying one.

Muscle Tension and Release

Lie down in a comfortable spot. Start by taking a slow
deep breath. As you breathe in, tighten your muscles
and make your hands into fists. When you breathe out,
loosen your muscles and relax your fingers. Hold and
tighten for about ten seconds and then release for about
ten seconds. Feel the difference between straining
and relaxing.

Progressive relaxation is when you relax each body
part one after another until you feel totally relaxed. Start
with your toes and tell them to relax. Move up to your
feet, then your legs, hips, stomach, hands, arms, chest,
lungs, shoulders, neck, chin, mouth, eyes, and head.
Each time you ascend your body, tell each body part to
relax. Take deep breaths until your whole body relaxes.

Rhythmic Breathing

You can do this lying down, or if you prefer, in a cross-
legged sitting position. Relax your body. It may help to
close your eyes and imagine a beautiful scene or to clear
your thoughts of all things so you can concentrate
strictly on your breathing. If you decide to keep your
eyes open, look at a distant object or, if you are at home,
stare into candlelight. Breathe in through your nose and
hold your breath for a count of ten. Let go of the air

45

slowly, counting to ten, through your mouth. Relax into your deep breathing and try to clear your mind. Feel yourself go limp every time you slowly breathe out. Work your time up to approximately ten minutes. When you are finished, slowly count to three, open your eyes, and come back to the present moment.

Autogenic Breathing
Autogenic breathing combines deep breathing with imagery for extremely effective stress relief. Start in a relaxed position, preferably lying down. Start deep rhythmic breathing. When you are relaxed and have found a comfortable breathing rhythm, visualize yourself on a sunny beach. The sun is warming you. Feel the warmth of the sun caress your skin, radiate into your muscles, and into your bones. Feel the soft, gentle breeze touch your body. Now imagine you are being gently cradled and the warmth relaxes your body more and more deeply. Now listen to the ebb of your breath. Say to yourself "warm" as the breath comes in and "deeply" as the breath goes out. Really try to feel the warmth in your body as the breath comes in and the feeling of being deeply relaxed as the breath goes out. Stay in the imagery of the beach until you feel relaxed.

Biofeedback
Biofeedback helps you have control over your body functions such as heart rate, blood pressure, and muscle tension. A biofeedback machine senses when your body

becomes tense. The machine then lets you know in some way, often using a flashing light, that you are experiencing stress. The machine also emits a signal when you are in a relaxed state. The goal is for you to be able to learn how to relax without the assistance of the machine. Ask someone at the hospital to refer you to a biofeedback specialist.

Imagery
Both visualization and imagery increase your sense of self-control and help you maintain a positive mind-set. Imagery is like self-hypnosis. First, find a comfortable position. Begin to breathe rhythmically. Imagine a white light of healing energy starting at your toes. When you see the white light, imagine as you breathe in that this healing energy is traveling to the parts of your body that feel pain or need energizing. When you breathe out, imagine the bad air and pain leaving your body. Continue to breathe, repeating "in with the good air" and "out with the bad air."

Visualization
Visualization is similar to imagery. Again, find a comfortable position either lying down or sitting up. Create an inner picture or imagine a scene that represents the battle between your cancer and your chemotherapy. Some people use images of rockets, dynamite, machine guns, or bombs blasting away those cancer cells. Some people imagine knights in armor, dinosaurs, ninjas, or warriors fighting the cancer cells.

47

The idea is to try to visualize the cancer cells being destroyed. You might also try a more soothing visualization exercise like the following.

The weeks have been chaotic but you are now safe on a train. You sink deeply into the luxury of the seat cushions. You glance out the window. The sun is setting, and red and purple clouds dot the painted sky. The light is about to fade, but you can still see the majestic mountains silhouetted against the sky. The low, rocking motion of the train blankets all other sounds. You sink more deeply into the seat. You have no problems to solve and nothing to think about as the train carries you into the sunset. It holds you, it rocks you, and it keeps you safe and warm inside.

Hypnosis

There are clinics and doctors that specialize in hypnotic techniques that help relieve pain, discomfort, and stress. Hypnosis allows you to enter a trancelike state and helps reduce your discomfort and anxiety. Ask your doctor or someone at the hospital to recommend a good therapist.

You can also engage in self-hypnosis. Close your eyes and feel your eyelids getting heavy. Take a deep breath, and as you exhale, feel your body relaxing. Use a cue word like "peace" and repeat this word to yourself as you exhale to deepen the relaxation. Now begin to focus on parts of your body. Tell yourself that your legs are becoming heavier and heavier and more and more relaxed. When you feel heaviness in your legs, concentrate on your arms. Again tell your arms that they are getting heavier and heavier and more and more relaxed.

Now concentrate on your face. Tell yourself that your forehead is becoming smooth and relaxed, now your cheeks are becoming smooth and relaxed. Now focus on your jaw. Open and close your mouth, and tell your jaw to become loose and relaxed. Now turn your attention to your neck and shoulders. Tell your shoulders to relax and droop. Take a slow breath in and relax your neck and shoulders. Take another breath in and relax your chest, stomach, and back. As you exhale, deepen the relaxation to your full torso.

Now it's time to go to a special place. It could be a beach, a resort, a park, or a room, but some place where you always feel loved and safe. Your special place can be a real or a magical place that you have conjured up. In a moment you will be there. Imagine reaching your special place by going down a flight of stairs, or a forest path, or a sandy beach. In ten steps you will be there.

With each step you grow more and more deeply relaxed, feeling peaceful and safe as you move to your special place. Now you will grow even more relaxed, counting each step: ten, nine, eight, seven, six, five, four, three, two, one, zero. You have arrived. You can repeat something like this over and over: "I am feeling stronger every day. I can relax through my chemotherapy treatments. The treatments are making me healthy. The cancer is dying. The treatments are killing it. I feel strengthened by the love of my friends and family. I can relax and let the chemotherapy work."

After you have repeated this suggestion a number of times, you can bring yourself back to normal conscious-ness. Count from one to ten. At number five, tell yourself that you are becoming more and more alert, refreshed, and awake. Around number nine, open your eyes. Enjoy the feeling of relaxation before you stand up.

Family

As we have discussed, the advent of cancer and chemotherapy treatments takes an emotional toll not only on the patient but also on his or her family and loved ones. It may also be frightening for a family member, especially a child, to watch a loved one undergo chemotherapy. Although chemotherapy helps patients fight cancer, during the process, patients look anything but improved. Family members look at their loved one and see total exhaustion, vomiting, loss of hair, and other side effects.

Siblings may resent the amount of attention paid to their brother or sister. Parents may tell them repeatedly, "We do not have any time for you right now." Young children may be unconsciously wishing their loved one would die so that the attention can be drawn back to them. Young chil-dren and teens may start acting out and throw tantrums, or experience night terrors and insomnia.

Younger siblings may also experience anxiety stemming from an irrational fear that cancer is contagious. More mature siblings may sense their own mortality. They may be concerned that they, too, will develop cancer later in life. They may feel anxious and frightened because their loved one may die. They may feel guilty because they are healthy.

Parents of a child with cancer may experience feelings of guilt as well. As Janet, whose son had leukemia as a child, explains, "I didn't feel guilty . . . at first. It wasn't until weeks after the diagnosis of leukemia that I felt overwhelming guilt: 'Why hadn't I noticed how sick Jeremy was? A new baby was no excuse.' My son has now grown into a tall, handsome boy; his fourteenth birthday approaches. I know I nag him too much. Perhaps it's time to back off and remind myself: 'He could have died.' Perhaps it's time to let him live his life."

Lending a Hand

Teens undergoing chemotherapy need to have the support of their family and friends. Sometimes the treatments go on for years. While initially patients receive support, after a time the support often thins. It is important that chemotherapy patients and their immediate family receive support throughout the entire process. Children, teens, and adults that we interviewed who were undergoing chemotherapy suggested some ways that people can help.

- ➣ Take care of the other children at home.

- ➣ Clean the apartment or house.

- ➣ Prepare meals for the rest of the family.

⮑ Offer to grocery shop for the rest of the family.

⮑ Send occasional notes expressing good wishes.

⮑ Relieve the caretaking parent at the hospital so the parent can attend to some of his or her own needs.

⮑ Ask the family how you can genuinely help.

⮑ Share your favorite CDs with the patient.

⮑ Read a short story to the patient.

⮑ Tolerate moods and silences.

⮑ Try not to act frightened by the side effects of chemotherapy.

⮑ Go shopping for a wig with your friend before the chemotherapy treatments.

⮑ Buy him or her the latest style in hat or head covering.

When children and teens are ill, they sometimes regress to a seemingly more immature stage. Many teenagers need an object like a stuffed toy or even their old baby blanket to comfort them. These objects are very therapeutic. One teen we interviewed took her musical backpack, which was in the shape of an animal, every-where she went. It was there before her operation and there when she woke up. It was there during her chemotherapy treatments. And it was also there when she finally returned home. Regardless of the method they use, people undergoing chemotherapy need to focus on themselves, their side effects, and their emotional highs and lows.

Patients' Stories

Cancer affects all age groups, and chemotherapy is used to treat young and old alike. The following are true stories of young people and an adult who have all endured chemotherapy. As these stories reveal, it is important for patients to have someone act as their advocate; someone the patient trusts who can ask questions when he or she feels weak. It is also very important for patients to empower themselves with as much information as possible about their cancer and their treatments.

Amanda, Age Fifteen

When you look back at your life, you are always look-ing for signs or indications that cancer cells were in your body. I had chronic nosebleeds. Could that have been the start of my cancer?

As a child, I was a creative writer and on the honor roll at school. When I was thirteen, it seems like overnight, I developed scoliosis, a curvature of the

*spine. I went to the doctor. He became very con-
cerned because I was also complaining of recurring
migraine headaches, dizzy spells, nausea, and vomiting. He arranged for an MRI (magnetic resonance
imaging), a type of CAT scan, to find out if there was
anything seriously wrong with me.*

*After he read the results, the doctor sent me directly
to Sick Children's Hospital. There was a tumor in the
back of my brain. A brain tumor! We were all in a state
of shock. The doctor told my mother that he was
unsure if it was malignant or benign. The hospital
admitted me right away, as there was fluid surrounding
the tumor—this was dangerous!*

*Six days later, I was operated on. Mom tells me
waiting for the doctor to come out of surgery was the
longest seven hours she spent in her life. The doctor
finally came out to tell her the news. The tumor was
the size of a large orange and had spread into the
ventricles. They could not remove the whole thing as
that would result in further brain damage.*

*After the operation, I discovered that my balance,
speech, and swallowing were affected. The worst
part was that some neurological damage had
occurred and I was left with facial paralysis. The
pathologist eventually informed me that the tumor
was malignant. That meant I had cancer.*

*I was very heavily sedated, and my mother had to
handle everything. The oncologist talked to Mom
and my grandmother. They were told that I had to
undergo ten courses of chemotherapy.*

*Everything was explained to me. Mom felt that she
had built a life of trust between us, and she wanted to*

maintain that trust when discussing my treatment. Mom was told that my treatment would take a long time. She left her job so she could devote herself to taking care of and advocating for me. I was extremely happy that Mom was there every day, as I could not handle the day-to-day events at the hospital without her. I relied heavily on her care.

Before even starting chemotherapy, right after the surgery, I had severe light sensitivity. I wanted to be in darkness all the time. I was very weak and complained bitterly of the pain in the back of my neck, due to my incision.

Each cancer is treated with a protocol unique for that type of cancer. They started me with a protocol called ICE. ICE was the first letter for each of the drugs they used in my protocol: Ifosfamide, Carboplatin, and Etoposide. I was to be treated with two courses of ICE, followed by thirty sessions of radiation directed at my spine and head, and another eight courses of chemotherapy.

When the first course of chemotherapy started, my mom was given pamphlets that explain the side effects of each drug. The pamphlets explained both short-term and long-term effects. Along with the ICE protocol, I also had to take drugs to protect my vital organs, like my liver and kidneys. My blood had to be constantly tested. White blood cells, platelets . . . everything drops after chemotherapy treatments.

Because of the operation, I started developing seizures, but it was imperative that I continue with the chemotherapy despite the side effects from the operation. After the first round of chemotherapy, I lost my hair and had sores in my mouth. I was scared when my hair fell out. I also had to take medication to control my seizures.

After the first chemotherapy treatment, I was allowed to go home. I stayed only one day. I had a high fever and was readmitted to the hospital. The next round of chemotherapy started. I was an inpatient and really was not aware of what was going on around me. An infection had developed around my incision and I ended up with meningitis. They had to insert a shunt (a bypass created surgically to permit flow from one region to another) to drain the fluid from around my brain. I was a very, very sick girl!

They changed the chemotherapy protocol four times because the ICE drugs were too strong. The next set of drugs were not strong enough. One set was so strong the drugs almost killed me. To this day, I do not know if it was the combination of all the drugs or one or more of the protocols that sent me into remission. All I do know is that each time I have an MRI, the residual tumor is smaller, and it is now the size of a hazelnut. The spine continues to be clear. I live for the day the MRI will show no tumor at all!

From all the chemotherapy drugs, my taste buds changed. I could not eat pizza for a whole year, also nothing with sauce or gravy. I do not know why. Maybe because of one of the memories of the drugs.

I am home now. I had cancer at the age of thirteen and I still have to undergo a number of surgeries to help alleviate the facial paralysis and, of course, my scoliosis. How does one go through all of this? My mom was there. She shared her inordinate strength *with me. She is also my memory. She kept a diary at all times. On every page she recorded my side effects, my pain, and my road to recovery. She was there to help keep me going.*

One time I told my mom I could not face the pain anymore and I wanted to go to heaven. My mom told me that she could not live without me and got the nurse, under the doctor's orders, to up my morphine. I remember my mom would read to me, especially sto-ries from Chicken Soup for the Teenage Soul.

When I finally got home from the hospital, we moved to a new apartment. My mom has painted a scene from an exotic place like France and Italy and Mexico on the walls of each room in our apartment. She is painting a skylight on the ceiling so together we will always be able to look out at the blueness of the sky and dream. She has created an oasis of beauty for me inside.

She is a beautiful woman who loves me so much that I have survived. We share the same dream. We both hope that each and every day I will continue to get strong and healthy.

Leukemia

Leukemia is cancer of the blood and bone marrow. Specifically, leukemia is a cancer in the tissue of bones or bone marrow, where the body manufactures both red and white blood cells. In fact, the bone marrow replaces all our blood once every twenty days. Each second, bone marrow produces more than ten million blood cells. At the same time, ten million other blood cells die. The bone marrow maintains cell count equilibrium.

Blood cell production in the bone marrow follows precise rules yet adapts quickly to all conditions in the body. If an infection is present, the bone marrow produces more infection-fighting white cells so the body is better equipped to fight germs. Once the infection is under control, the number of white blood cells produced drops to a normal level.

Unfortunately, in a body stricken with leukemia, as the number of cancer cells increases, healthy bone marrow is crowded out. The leukemic cells become so numerous they fill the bone cavity, making it almost impossible for healthy cells to develop. The lack of these healthy cells results in symptoms associated with leukemia: anemia, hemorrhaging, and infection.

With the onset of leukemia, cancerous cells multiply faster than normal cells. Soon there are so many cancerous cells that the white blood cells cannot fight off germs. This leaves the body more vulnerable to disease and infection. When the bone marrow cannot make enough red blood cells to carry oxygen throughout the body, a person feels exhausted. The cancer cells also overcrowd the stem cells that enable the body to stop bleeding. The body therefore bleeds and bruises very easily.

Leukemia can be divided into two main groups: chronic and acute. Chronic leukemia occurs mostly in adults. Acute leukemia is more common among young people. There are two subgroups of acute leukemia:

acute lymphoblastic leukemia (ALL) and acute non-lymphoblastic leukemia (ANLL). ALL accounts for 70 to 80 percent of cases in children.

A doctor can easily diagnose leukemia by examining bone marrow. The preferred treatment is chemotherapy. These treatments are very difficult, particularly in the first three months. The maintenance period, which can continue for a period of two to three years, is easier to bear.

Richard, Age Thirteen

I was only six when I became sick, but I do remember being carefree and I loved playing soccer. I was in first grade and I was very tired. I didn't have the stamina to do activities like I always did and my nose bled daily. At first, Mom thought it was a persistent cold virus. She then thought I might have a platelet disorder like my older brother had. Mom took me to the doctor. He did some tests. The doctor was a family friend and we soon received a call from the doctor's wife. She was very upset and told my mom to come to the office to talk.

When we got to the doctor's office, he kept reading the paper in front of him. He did not say anything for at least five minutes. "Blasts, an overabundance in the blood," he said. Blasts are young cells found solely in the bone marrow. Their presence in the blood usually indicates infection.

Mom understood that blasts meant leukemia, but she did not believe it. Mom thought the doctor was all wrong and she hoped that at the hospital she would hear a completely new story. It was 1992, the Toronto Blue Jays had won the World Series, the horns were blaring, and I was on the way to the hospital. I was admitted right away and diagnosed with leukemia.

They took a sample from my bone marrow to find out what type of leukemia I had. I had ALL, the most common type. My blast count was so high that I was given the protocol for high-risk leukemia patients. I know I was told about chemotherapy and the side effects, but looking back now, I really can't remember. Mom said I asked a lot of questions. I apparently wanted to know all about the drugs I was taking. I wanted to know why I had to take that particular drug. The drugs made me very sleepy. Mom and sometimes Dad stayed overnight with me; my two brothers were at home.

On the seventh day of chemotherapy, I continued to vomit. I took some Gravol, hoping it would help alleviate this side effect, but the nausea continued. I can say this: Chemotherapy is pretty powerful. I remember taking a drug and it turned my urine red. My hair did fall out but I grew accustomed to it. The sores in my mouth hurt a lot and my stomach felt awful.

I was lucky that after two weeks of chemotherapy, I went into remission. That meant for two years I was on maintenance. Every two weeks, I had blood work done, and smaller rounds of chemotherapy were administered. The nausea and vomiting continued. For two years, my breakfast ended up in the toilet. The Gravol would make me feel tired so it was hard to go to school.

I never felt sorry for myself. I persevered. I accepted what happened and what was happening to me. I never *doubted that I was going to get better in the long run. I was strong emotionally and accepting. They would say, "Tomorrow you need to go for your spinal tap." I would then ask if I could have a toy after it was over.*

I had a port (a small plastic or metal container surgically placed under the skin, through which blood and fluids can enter or leave the body) and just put up with it. They put me on steroids, which made me gain weight in my upper body, and prednisone, a drug that altered my moods. I was doing real well, and for three years (ages eight to eleven), I did not need any treatment.

Unfortunately, when I was eleven I had a relapse. I was immediately hospitalized and they tried a different type of protocol. I was on a thirty-six-hour drip of chemotherapy plus more drugs to protect my body from the chemotherapy drugs. They were now looking for a bone marrow transplant donor. This would save my life. The doctors searched the bone marrow registry, but they could not find a match. My brothers matched each other but not me.

Finally, after seven months, a match was found, but in the end it was not a good match. My father was not a perfect match, but since we were running out of time, we went with him. A bone marrow transplant is an intense and painful process. My mother wished she could take the pain for me. She said, "If I knew the bone marrow transplant would be so difficult on you, I wouldn't have had you go through it. Maybe I am being selfish trying to hang on to you for a little while longer." I told her, "Don't ever say that! I'm glad I am here."

It's funny. After getting my dad's bone marrow, I also developed his sleep disorder. When my own bone marrow started to grow back, I no longer experienced his sleep disorder.

I have just graduated from the eighth grade, and I am looking forward to starting high school in September. One thing the chemotherapy has affected is my memory. At times I just can't remember things. I've learn to joke about it. I feel that I have survived because of my strong will. I am a strong believer that your mind plays a big part in how long you exist. It has been one year from my transplant, and guess what? I am doing just fine!

Chris, Age Twelve

My family was no stranger to leukemia. My cousin died from it when he was only four years old. Could such a disease strike twice in one family? I was only seven when I started feeling miserable. I had a cough that did not go away. I was crying all the time. I was becoming pale and feeling drained.

Six months earlier, my parents had asked the doctor about my weight loss and the loss of my appetite. The doctor thought that I was in the midst of a growth spurt and told them not to worry. The glands around my neck were swollen, and my parents continued to worry.

The doctor told my parents to have my blood tested. On a Saturday morning at a private clinic, my blood was taken. Sunday morning, the pediatrician called. She suspected leukemia; I needed to be treated right away as I was very anemic. My parents felt like *they were living in a nightmare. They figured it was a one-in-a-million chance that this could happen in the same family again.*

My parents took me down to the hospital. There, the doctor ordered more blood work. I remember being terrified of needles. As long as my parents distracted me, I was fine. That Sunday afternoon, the oncologist confirmed the diagnosis: It was leukemia. After further testing of the bone marrow, I was diagnosed with ALL (acute lymphoblastic leukemia).

I was told that I was going to be put on a drug protocol for three years. We were told that 75 to 80 percent of children were completely cured. Immediately, I started chemotherapy treatments. I was told that I would lose my hair, gain some weight, feel nauseous and tired, and that I could develop sores in my mouth. As I would encounter stomach upsets, I was also given Gravol.

One drug they administered, Vincristine, made me feel achy. I felt as though my body was being trapped. All I really wanted was not to feel the needles. I was so scared of them.

In the operating room, the doctors inserted a port. They always used a cream that would freeze my skin so I would not feel the pain. I was given a number of drugs different days of the week, for one month. I finally came home as an outpatient but visited the clinic every day. I had minimal hair loss after the first treatment, but my hair texture changed. My curly hair went straight. My sense of smell became acute. I hated hospital food, the look and the smell of it.

I was lucky I tolerated the drugs very well. I was not too nauseous and did not experience the typical stomach problems. When I was about nine years old, my platelet level became so low that I had to have a transfusion. Only one donor had my partic- ular platelets. In the course of the three years, I had to be readmitted to the hospital only twice.

I was scared throughout this whole ordeal. My family worried about me constantly. Nothing was the same; nothing seemed normal! There were a lot of prayers said in the family, from across the seas, and in town.

During my third and fourth sessions of chemotherapy, I stayed in the hospital. One drug even turned my skin yellow. I was in remission for three years. I completed grades three to five at school, but then my blood count became low. I had a relapse; ALL once again. It was rec- ommended that I undergo a bone marrow transplant.

With chemotherapy treatments alone, the chance of remission would be less than 10 percent, but with a bone marrow transplant, the chances increased to 45 or 50 percent. The whole family was tested. My sister Jessica turned out to be the perfect match. I had to go for chemotherapy as well as radiation treatments before the transplant. My bone marrow needed to be completely clear of all bad cells in order to receive my sister's healthy and clean cells.

As I grew older, I came to understand my illness. I did not feel sorry for myself; maybe I did, but I did not admit it to myself. I was angry. I felt like life sucks. I thought, "Do I have to do this all over again?" All I wanted was to be with my friends. In the back of my mind, I wondered if I would die. One day, I asked the hospital staff. They told me, "No, don't worry, but things can happen."

My sister's bone marrow saved my life. The whole ordeal of me being in and out of the hospital was very difficult for her emotionally. At times I know she felt that all the attention was on me; she felt abandoned. Nevertheless, she did give me the greatest gift: a new life.

Throughout my sickness, my parents comforted me. Both Mom and Dad spent time at the hospital. I could always depend on them. It is summer now, and I am going off to camp for two weeks. Everyone still worries, but right now I am looking forward to being just a regular kid!

Ovarian Cancer

Ovarian cancer is a malignancy in one or both ovaries. The ovaries are the two almond-sized glands on either side of a woman's uterus. The American Cancer Society estimates that 25,400 new cases of ovarian cancer are diagnosed annually in the United States. Each year, an estimated 14,500 women die from the disease. Although ovarian cancer may metastasize, or spread, anywhere in the body, it commonly spreads to nearby organs such as the stomach and intestines.

On average, a woman has a 1.4 percent chance of being diagnosed with ovarian cancer in her lifetime. Women with a close female relative like a mother, sister, or daughter who has ovarian cancer have a 7 percent chance of developing the disease. Studies of Japanese women exposed to the atomic bomb in World War II revealed almost twice the expected number of ovarian cancer cases. Other research has examined the link between ovarian cancer and fat intake.

66

The disease seldom produces symptoms until it begins to spread. Such symptoms include an enlarged abdomen, persistent abdominal discomfort, indigestion, nausea, vomiting, weight loss, diarrhea, constipation, and uterine bleeding that does not correspond to a woman's period. The primary treatment is removal of one or both of the ovaries and, in more advanced stages, a combination of surgery and chemotherapy.

Alice, Age Eighteen

I guess you could say I was an all-around athlete and honor student before I became sick. I played basketball and volleyball, and won many medals in track. I was fifteen, in the eighth grade, and I had just won the female athlete of the year award. I was valedictorian at my graduation.

After this exciting time, my family and I traveled to Montreal, Canada, to stay with friends. I had severe abdominal pains and was constantly vomiting. My mother quickly took me to the doctor to see what was wrong. The doctor thought it might just be anxiety from graduation and all. We came back home to Toronto, but I continued to vomit and was experiencing severe diarrhea.

Mom was very worried and took me straight to the hospital. If the symptoms continued, the doctor said, come back to the hospital. They gave me medication and sent me home, and I was fine.

Two years later, in the fall, at age seventeen, the attack started all over again. This time I thought it might just be stomach flu, but Mom insisted that the

67

doctor examine me anyway. When the doctor asked about my medical history, I told her what had occurred two years ago.

Since the summer months, my stomach had been growing. It was hard when I touched it. I was embarrassed about my stomach so I did not tell anyone, including my mom. The doctor decided not to take any chances.

She ordered an ultrasound. The ultrasound showed a large cyst on my left ovary. The doctor told my mom and me to go straight down to the hospital. More tests again. I was very scared; I really did not know what to expect! They gave me a blood test to find out the levels of my alpha-fetoprotein. Mom knew they were looking for indications of cancer. Mom was told that the normal level was around five to ten, but my level was 1,300—extremely high.

They sent me home pending surgery. The word "cancer" was never once mentioned to me directly. Mom is a nurse, and she followed everything that was happening to me very closely. She kept a diary right from the beginning. I told my mom, "You have to stay strong for me, and I will stay strong for you."

The operation took over four hours. Our worst fears were confirmed: It was cancer. The tumor and ovary were removed. The tumor was encapsulated, which means there was no leakage; the cancer had not spread. We were referred to an oncologist and discussed treatment options. The oncologist decided against chemotherapy at that time.

After the operation, the doctor checked the level of protein in my blood. The first week, there was a drop from 1,300 to 700, then during the next two weeks, a drop to 425, then 300. It finally leveled off at twenty. Then it started to rise again to 120. It was decided that three rounds of chemotherapy would be administered.

A team from the hospital, including my oncologist, nurse, and social worker, all came into my room to answer any questions about chemotherapy and explain the side effects to me. They told me that I would lose my hair and that the drugs could make me sick with nausea and vomiting. The social worker gave me the telephone number for a wig shop. I had chemotherapy treatments in the hospital for five days, then was out for three weeks, and then returned again for the next round.

I had a PICC line inserted a couple of days before the first round. I wished I did not have to go through it all. I had nausea and vomiting, and developed sores in my mouth immediately. When I got home, I couldn't walk all of a sudden. I was rushed to the emergency room. An extra dose of chemotherapy had caused this paralysis. I couldn't walk for a couple of days.

The chemotherapy made me very sick and tired. I lost all my energy. As blood counts drop after chemotherapy, risk of infection increases. I could not go into crowds because of fear of infection. After the second round of chemotherapy, my hair fell out.

After the third round of chemotherapy, another scan revealed a cyst in my other ovary. Mom went to church and prayed and prayed. I decided that I was not going to have my other ovary removed. Mom and the doctor both disagreed with my decision. I told them if they did *another scan and I could see the cyst, I would agree. I finally agreed with everyone; I would undergo the surgery. Before the second surgery, the doctor thought the cancer had spread; she saw something in my head with the CT scan. Mom insisted on an MRI, which revealed that the cancer had not spread.*

Unfortunately, both my ovaries were removed. After my operation, I was informed that the second ovary was not cancerous. Sometimes I am angry with these doctors for removing my last ovary; at other times I know they did it with my best interest in mind. I am upset that I can never have children of my own. I also have to take medication all my life to keep my estrogen levels up.

Now I go for frequent checkups, and I am doing fine. I really relied on support from my friends, family, church, hospital, and teachers. I want to be a pediatrician when I am older, so I can help children, too.

Lymphoma

A lymphoma is a tumor in the lymphatic glands. There are two distinct types of lymphoma: Hodgkin's and non-Hodgkin's lymphoma. The presence of swollen glands in the neck or armpit is often one of the first signs of Hodgkin's lymphoma. Symptoms associated with the disease are weight loss, high and irregular fever, perspiring at night, and itchiness. It is usually treated with radiation therapy and, in more advanced stages, with chemotherapy and radiation. Approximately 80 percent of patients can hope to recover.

Non-Hodgkin's lymphoma consists of malignant tumors; the cells are derived from lymphocytes. Leukemia begins in the bone marrow cells, and non-Hodgkin's lymphoma begins in the lymph glands. The treatment is the same as that for leukemia and consists primarily of chemotherapy and radiation treatment. Approximately 80 percent of patients experience complete remission, depending on the extent to which the tumor has spread.

Natalie, Age Seventeen

At my high school graduation, my mom joined me onstage for an emotional embrace and said, "I am so happy to see her graduate, there were times I didn't know we'd get to this day." I had been out of school an entire year, and my mom had sacrificed so much in order to pay the tuition for my final year.

But I am jumping ahead; let's go back to when I was just fourteen.

I loved to write and constantly jotted things down in my journal. I have always been an 'A' student with lots and lots of friends. I loved basketball, and people said I was always on the go. It was 6:00 PM and I was on the way to basketball practice when I started to feel dizzy and nauseous. I passed out.

My brother took me to the office and they called an ambulance to take me to the hospital. They ran all sorts of tests on me. They thought I had a bowel obstruction (blocked bowel). I was steadily losing weight so they went ahead and performed emergency surgery. They removed eight inches of my bowel. My small intestine had wrapped inside my large intestine.

Two weeks later, we were asked to see an oncologist. Mom went with me. I did not even know at that time what an oncologist was. He said he just got the pathology report, and the part they removed from me showed that I had cancer. I turned to him and asked, "You sure you're talking about me?" I was in shock. He said that everything was okay now and hopefully the cancer would not return. I was diagnosed with non-Hodgkin's lymphoma.

Every two months, I visited the oncologist, and he told me repeatedly that everything was looking good. I was going every three months when I started to get pains in my side and stomach. They injected radiation dye to show the "hot spots" in my body. You could see right on the screen that I had tumors in my lower abdomen.

The doctors recommended that I undergo chemotherapy because the original surgery had not gotten rid of the cancer cells. I then went to Children's Hospital, where they did more tests. They gave me a pamphlet, and I watched a video on chemotherapy. I was told I might lose weight depending on the protocol. I did not know what questions to ask. I was overwhelmed!

I reacted very, very badly to the second round of chemotherapy. My blood counts were so low that I needed a blood transfusion. My mom asked the doctor how bad my condition was. He said, "Put it this way: If she stubs her toe on the bed, she could bleed to death." My blood counts were so low that my body could not fight fast enough. I had to have my platelets transfused. My mom said I was so weak that she had to pick me up to go to the bathroom.

72

Unfortunately, I was unique in how I reacted to some of the chemotherapy drugs. One drug that supposedly had little side effects sent me into convulsions; with another that had many side effects, I was fine. My heart rate dropped so low that they put me on a heart monitor. My kidneys started to fail. Mom told me I was hooked up to everything. I had no idea how deathly ill I was. They gave me morphine, but that gave me itchy skin and hallucinations.

The chemotherapy had a number of side effects. At the hospital, they said I must be one of the unluckiest kids when it came to side effects. I was exhausted and slept all the time. I vomited and had sores in my mouth all the way down to my throat. I lost every hair on my whole body! One drug made my heels and fingers feel like I had pins and needles in them.

I thought I might die. I asked the oncologist my chances, and he said that I had an 80 percent chance of survival. With the help of my mom and my brother, I knew I was going to fight this thing!

After my fourth round of chemotherapy, I came home. Mom had a nurse stay with me so she could go back to work. I then got a blood infection in my PICC line and was rushed back to the hospital. I had another bowel obstruction. I had many surgeries and over 400 needles in my arms and legs. I begged them to tell me when this would all end. Their only response: "When you get better."

I kept a positive attitude throughout the whole terrible ordeal. If I had let it get me down, I might have given up the fight, but I did not. I was told I was on my deathbed four times. I would do it all over again

because it saved my life. It was a hard road to climb, but it has been two years and I am still cancer free!
Now, I volunteer my time; I talk to kids about cancer. I just received the Governor General Award of Ontario, Canada, for my good deeds. I want to do something good with my life, and this year I will be studying to become a nurse specializing in cancer. Maybe, just maybe, I will publish my journal that tells how I survived. I always love a happy ending, don't you?

Colorectal Cancer

Colorectal cancer is a malignancy of the large intestine (the lower portion of the intestinal tract), which consists of the colon and rectum. It is most common in the section closest to the rectum. Colon and rectal cancers are the third most common of all cancers, as well as the third most frequent cause of cancer death in men and women.

A family history of colorectal cancer, polyps (growths in the lining of the colon), or inflammatory bowel disease are also risk factors. Some signs of colorectal cancer are blood in the stool, persistent constipation, severe diarrhea, abdominal pain, or unexplained weight loss. Colonoscopy, the process that allows the doctor to view the entire length of the large intestine, is recommended for people at high risk and those over the age of fifty. The primary treatment for colorectal cancer is surgery to remove the tumor, followed by radiation and/ or chemotherapy.

Susan, Age Forty-Seven

I was forty-four and had just celebrated my twenty-fifth wedding anniversary with my husband. I was feeling happy and healthy. I had four wonderful children and imagined a rosy future with my whole family. I wanted to lose weight, so I watched what I ate and started jogging. I had lost ten pounds in one year and was feeling on top of the world. The doctor had put me on iron pills, as my iron level was constantly low.

We had just recently gotten a puppy, and it was like having another infant in the house. I was starting to get pains in my gut, just below my belly button. I asked the vet if I had caught something from the puppy, like worms. At the same time, my husband was having difficulties at work. He decided to look for another job. Needless to say, there was stress in our household.

I mentioned the pain to my friend who was a nurse. She encouraged me to follow up with my family doctor. I was having many bowel movements and thought because of all the stress in the house I was suffering from "irritable bowel syndrome." I was taking four to six Advils (ibuprofen) a day for the pain. I thought if I ate less, I would have less pain. I then started to lose weight. I finally went to see the family doctor. She did not send me to a specialist. She told me to eat more bran and thought the pain was from the iron pills I was presently taking. I was now up to ten Advils a day to ease the pain.

One day, I was helping out at my children's school and had to leave to take the puppy out for a walk. I

75

ran to the bathroom and had bloody diarrhea. I must have lost almost a liter of blood. I was in a state of shock. I just hoped it would go away. I telephoned the family doctor and made an appointment for the next day. Then I had another episode and got in touch with the doctor personally. She said it was probably a bleeding hemorrhoid and not to worry, to just come in first thing in the morning. I was very shaky and anxious, and feeling weak.

The next morning, the doctor sent me right over to have an emergency procedure to see if anything was wrong in my rectum. The GI (gastroenterologist) resident interviewed me, and based on my symptoms knew right away what was wrong with me. I could not go home. He could not believe the size of the blockage in my rectum. I had to have surgery. They were pretty sure I had cancer.

Colon cancer, how could it be? Most of my family had been cancer free. I drank lots of water, exercised regularly, ate properly—how could I have colon cancer? A couple of weeks later, I was operated on. My cancer was in stage three; one node was affected. Chemotherapy was a sure thing!

I received chemotherapy treatments as an out-patient. They injected a vein in my hand. They asked me if I wanted to have a Popsicle, ginger ale, or ice chips. I chose ice chips. They told me that they give patients something cold to eat in order to constrict the blood vessels. Therefore the drugs will be less likely to travel to noncancerous areas. To this day, I cannot have ice because it reminds me of my treatments!

The nurses were very good. They made sure that I received the correct protocol. They also wrote down how I was doing and what I said. I had to have a blood test before every treatment. The doctor wanted to make sure that my hemoglobin count was high enough for me to receive chemotherapy. The treatment lasted only about fifteen minutes. After my third and fourth treatments, I kept a bowl by my head to vomit into. Actually, as soon as I entered the hospital I would get waves of nausea. I thought it was a primal kind of thing. My body did not want those harsh drugs in it!

I was strong; I wanted to do whatever it took to stay alive. I wanted to live and I just wanted to make sure the cancer never came back. Before my chemotherapy treatments, I cut my hair short. From the drugs, I lost a lot of hair; it really thinned out—my eyebrows, too. My skin color was more sallow. I felt very weak and tired. During my final treatment, I had an anxiety attack. I felt as if I was coming to the edge of an abyss. This was the final treatment and I had been proactive up to this point in time. I could not bear the thought of not doing something active to prevent the cancer from recurring.

The hardest thing for me was the thought of leaving my children without a mother. I had been told I had a 60 percent chance of survival. I did not tell my children or other family members. My husband was there for me and we cried together.

After all the treatments were complete, I asked the doctor, "What next?" Now, I have checkups every two to three months. I did ask the oncologist,

"Why me?" He answered, "The cell mutated and unfortunately yours grew." Now, I celebrate more, and I enjoy every good thing that comes along. I have been cancer free for over three years. I celebrate with champagne and toast the world with the words "To Life!"

Doctors' Stories

The following are true stories told by oncologists, doctors who specialize in the diagnosis and treatment of different types of cancers. You will encounter oncologists in the course of your own treatment or during your loved one's treatment. You may want to be an oncologist yourself one day.

Dr. Mark Greenberg, Pediatric Oncologist

Why did I want to be a pediatric oncologist? I always wanted to be an interventionist; I wanted to make a difference. It was important for me to work with families, to understand the whole physical and emotional picture. At first, I was going to get into infectious diseases. I set up a matrix, really a self-help graph, to discover what specialty was best for me to enter. Finally, I chose oncology, specifically treating children with cancer.

Oncology is a high-intensity field. You touch life and death day in and day out. As a result, those working in this field also have a high burnout rate.

A young couple came into the office with their child; the child had a brain tumor. I told them his chances for survival were good, but the child would require an operation and treatment.

The child was bright, and the surgery would affect him intellectually. The parents fell apart; they saw the dream of their child as a future professional fall apart. I told them the child may not grow up to be a surgeon but will live a satisfactory life.

It was important for them to understand that the dream for their child would have to be an altered dream, but they could still have a dream. One does not trash a dream; one reframes it. The child will have his own accomplishments and achievements in life. I could not sugarcoat the situation, but I could talk about other survivors. When appropriate, I give families hope and an understanding that there is a future.

I had a teenager come to the hospital who was an athlete and a violinist. She had to have her arm and leg amputated because of cancer. She would never play the violin again, but her life as an athlete flourished. Recently, she won a silver medal in the Para-Olympics.

Sometimes, when children are dying, parents want me to help their child stay alive until the next holiday, like Christmas. I tell them that Christmas is a concept and that they should make next Friday Christmas. It is a celebration, and the time to celebrate is now. There is no need to wait.

How do I tell children and teens about cancer and chemotherapy? I like to draw a verbal picture or analogy that helps me explain a concept. Patients often wonder why they need to take so many drugs.

I give the example of the baker. The baker requires yeast, flour, and water, then he or she mixes it, bakes it, and makes bread. If you lack any of these ingredients, you will not be able to make bread. In your body you have many cells, and they are constantly dividing and making multiple cells. If you block the water, the yeast, and the flour, the bread cannot be made. If the chemicals in chemotherapy are blocking the active ingredients in the cells, the cancer cannot continue to thrive. DNA cannot be made in the cancerous cell.

Although we block the cancerous cells from growing, unfortunately some normal cells can also be affected. That is why in the course of chemotherapy some healthy cells, like those affecting hair, will be affected and the hair will fall out.

I like to talk directly to a teen about his or her cancer and treatment. It is also good if the parents are involved as well. It is my job to provide them with a specific diagnosis. I want them to understand there are no secrets.

I may say something like, "We have now confirmed that you have cancer. The type of cancer is . . . Let me tell you about it. I want to tell you what the next move is and here is how we fix it. Lots of kids have gone through the treatment with good outcomes, but it is not an easy ride. Still, we get most kids through it."

It is also important how I relate to the patients. The children and parents watch my every body movement and facial expression when I have to tell them about the cancer and treatment. I realize that being told one has cancer and about the treatment for it evokes many emotions. I remember a teenager with cancer in his pelvis. I explained to him that once he had his operation, his body would be scarred.

He was very angry; he punched the wall and left the room to go to a shopping mall and hang out. I waited all day until he finally returned. He was scared that he would not have a normal life and girls would not find him appealing after he was disfigured from his surgery. I heard from him recently; he is twenty-seven, married, and has just completed his master's degree.

Sometimes during the course of the chemotherapy, teenagers will regress; they may need a stuffed toy or a favorite possession to take with them to their sessions. I try to make the treatments less scary for them. I try to let them have some feeling of control, like asking what finger they want me to prick.

Teens are very aware of self-image and fashion. Losing hair is a big issue. They do not want to look like they are sick. During the treatments, some teens like to be left alone, some like to plug into music, but most of all they want to get going and get out.

What are some questions teens ask? They all seem to focus on their hair and when it will grow back or if it will grow back at all. They seem to want to know if they will look different. Some ask about blood transfusions and the risk of infection. Some ask if they can infect others.

I have seen siblings feel guilty and wonder if they somehow caused the cancer. I have found that mothers tend to feel especially guilty; was there something, anything they should have done?

I try to educate and reassure patients and their family members. I tell them about feeling crappy, vomiting, hair loss, and a drug that turns the urine red. I tell them ways to cope with nausea. I do talk to teens about fertility and potency. High doses of drugs may affect a girl's period.

Many teens are overwhelmed at first. Initially they may not ask if the treatments will cure them or if they are going to die. I try to be both a friend and a doctor to my teen patients.

Breast Cancer

Breast cancer is a malignant tumor in the glandular tissues of the breast. Carcinomas (tumors) tend to destroy an increasing proportion of normal breast tissue over time and may spread or metastasize to other parts of the body. Breast cancer is unfortunately the most common cancer in women (men can be affected as well).

More than 80 percent of all breast cancers are first detected as unusual masses in the breast. These masses are detected through self-examination, a routine doctor checkup, or by mammography (an X ray of the breast). Removal of the cancerous tumor through surgery cures one-third of all breast cancers that are detected early.

Chemotherapy, or the administration of cancer-fighting drugs such as Taxol, has proven effective in destroying breast cancer cells that have spread to other organs. The five-year survival rate for American women diagnosed with localized breast cancer increased from 78 percent in the 1940s to 97 percent in the 1990s. If the cancer has spread to adjacent tissue, the five-year survival rate is 76 percent.

Dr. Ellen Warner, Oncologist

Ever since I was a little girl I wanted to find a cure for cancer. I became a doctor, as cancer doctors were needed in Israel, where I lived. When I left Israel, I moved to Canada. Here, I work with women and a few men in all stages of breast cancer. My patients are usually at least twenty-five years old, but I also work with younger women to test if they might be genetically predisposed to developing breast cancer.

Surgeons usually refer their breast cancer patients to me. The cancer and possibly the lymph nodes under the arm have already been removed by the time they come to see me. I look at the pathology report and the tumor, and discuss with the patients whether they may need chemotherapy.

I tell my patients that chemotherapy involves powerful drugs that can be taken intravenously or in pill form. Chemotherapy is a way to live longer, not a cure. It may decrease the reoccurrence of cancer by 30 percent.

Many of the women I deal with find the visible signs of being sick upsetting. Many have already lost a breast. For some, the loss devastates their self-image, and the thought of losing their hair to chemotherapy treatments can be doubly upsetting. Women also ask about the vomiting and nausea. There are good drugs on the market nowadays that help prevent these side effects, so it is rarely a problem. I tell my patients that their blood counts will drop and they may develop sores in their mouth, diarrhea, constipation, some weight gain, and fatigue.

Young women often ask about fertility. Some women will not compromise their fertility and will therefore refuse treatment. Older women usually want to know if the chemotherapy will cause early menopause.

Sometimes as doctors we advise breast cancer patients to undergo chemotherapy. We ask ourselves, should we prescribe chemotherapy as a preventive measure? We also wonder if a patient chose not to have chemotherapy, would there be a reoccurrence? One never really knows for sure. There is no 100 percent certain solution. I try hard to help and give the proper advice to all my patients.

Dr. Jeffrey Lipton, Oncologist

I received my Ph.D. in biochemistry and then went on to earn my medical degree. I did research on leukemia and went back to medical school to treat leukemia. There, I had the ideal opportunity to correlate biology and treatment. Research in leukemia allowed me to look at cell processes, particularly how cells grow. One can grow leukemia cells in a test tube. I can see how cells react to chemotherapy. I wanted to work with people, combining my interest *in research and patient care. I have been involved with treatment for over thirteen years.*

I keep very long hours. I will start work as early as 4:30 AM and come home as late as 8:00 PM. I usually work 80 to 100 hours a week.

Usually, another specialist refers his or her patient to me. A teenager usually arrives with other family members like parents, but not always. I ask the patient what he or she already knows and tell him or her what I know or at least what I suspect is going on. I tell the patient what I need to do to confirm the diagnosis and determine what to do if the body does not respond to treatment. I also review the prognosis or features of the disease, as not all leukemias are the same.

I try to educate the person. I tell my patient what he or she can expect without treatment. I may tell him or her that he or she will be undergoing intensive chemotherapy with the intent to cure.

Leukemia can be overwhelming for everybody, especially for teenagers. They may be cooped up in the hospital enduring side effects that last years, and their education may be affected. They may already be struggling to maintain a positive body image before entering the hospital, and with leukemia they have to deal with many emotional and physical changes.

Many teenagers receive support from their peers. If they are not so popular, treatment may be especially difficult for them. Some parents try to protect their teenager and do not give them all the information about his or her condition. I feel it is important that parents know that I am honest and that they can trust me. I find teens can be unforgiving if you lie. If I am recommending a risk, they need to be able to trust my judgment. If a teenage patient does not speak English, I consult an outside interpreter instead of a family member.

Teens often ask questions like can they go to a special event like a party or a prom? I sometimes have to give my teen patients a reality check. In other words, I might have to tell them that they may not be able to finish their exams or may have to drop out of university that year. I have found that teens rarely ask me if they are going to die. They may think it, but they don't ask.

I explain that chemotherapy is the use of toxic drugs designed to kill leukemia cells. Chemotherapy can affect normal cells, particularly faster growing cells like hair, gastro lining, and bone marrow. Chemotherapy treatment can vary, but usually the treatment lasts six to seven days continuously (depending on the type of leukemia and the drugs used).

The side effects can include feeling groggy, nauseous, mildly unwell, or horribly sick the whole time. Patients may run a continuous fever. Patients may even die from the treatment.

Nurses deal with a patient's day-to-day emotional stress. The nurses spend more time with the patient and can connect and talk with him or her. I often have less time to interact with a patient at length. I will sometimes bring in a patient who has already undergone a bone marrow transplant to talk to a new patient or recommend a psychologist or social worker.

Chemotherapy is protocol-driven. It is a drug cocktail, not a single drug. We try the best drugs first. If

*there is a relapse and no bone marrow transplant, the
eventuality could be death. In some cases, though, we
have been extremely successful.*

*I have the difficult job of doing bone marrow trans-
plants. There are only three doctors in our city who
perform the kind of transplant that I do. Nevertheless,
I enjoy what I do and am good at it.*

*I see each individual as a person, not as a disease.
Every once in a while, someone affects me deeply—if
the prognosis is bad, it can be devastating. I can't cure
everybody, but I usually can make them better for a
brief period of time. I love it when I have treated a kid
and later on in life he or she comes back and shows
me his or her own children.*

CONCLUSION

Cancer and chemotherapy often go hand in hand. If we
eliminate cancer we will eliminate the need for
chemotherapy. We are coming closer and closer to understanding why cells mutate. We may soon eliminate certain
cancers. Through research we will eventually gain a full
understanding of cancers and one day find a cure. In the
meantime, children, teens, and adults will undergo
chemotherapy and hopefully live long, productive lives.

According to researcher and author David Drum, "Eight
million Americans are alive today who have been diagnosed with cancer, including four million diagnosed within
the past five years. Sophisticated medical treatment is the

reason why most of these people are expected to survive and live normal life spans." It has not been easy for any of these cancer survivors, but they are here to remind us that the long, hard road of chemotherapy has been worth it. After all, they are here to tell their stories!

Although the world is full of suffering, it is also full of the overcoming of it.

—Helen Keller

Glossary

anemia   Condition of having too few red blood cells. Symptoms of anemia include feeling tired, weak, and short of breath.

benign tumor   A noncancerous tumor.

biopsy   Removal of body tissue for viewing under a microscope.

blasts   Young cells, the precursors of white cells, red cells, and platelets. Blasts are found solely in the bone marrow. Their presence in the blood is unusual; when detected, doctors look for serious infections like an inflammatory disease or leukemia.

blood count   The number of red blood cells, white blood cells, and platelets in a sample of blood. This is also called complete blood count (CBC).

bone marrow   The inner, spongy tissue of bones where blood cells are made.

cancer   A general term for more than 100 diseases in which abnormal cells grow out of control; a malignant tumor.

carcinogen   Any substance or agent that produces cancer.

carcinoma   A cancer that begins on the surface of certain organs. Carcinoma of the skin, or skin cancer, is among the most common forms.

catheter A small, thin, plastic tube that can be introduced into a vein, an artery, or any cavity from which liquid must be removed; it is also used to administer drugs.

cell The smallest living structure in an organism. Several cells grouped together and fulfilling a very special function form an organ.

central-venous catheter A special thin, flexible tube placed in a large vein. It remains there for as long as it is needed to deliver and withdraw fluids.

chemotherapy The treatment of cancer with (often toxic) chemical substances.

chronic A condition that is characterized by long duration and frequent recurrence.

clot A clot is formed of platelets, red blood cells, and proteins. Its main function is to stop hemorrhaging.

colonoscopy An examination of the inner lining of the rectum and colon with a flexible, lighted instrument.

CT (or CAT) scan A series of detailed pictures of areas inside the body created by a computer linked to an X-ray machine. Also called computed tomography (CT) scan or computed axial tomography (CAT) scan.

diagnosis Confirmation that cancer (or other condition) is present or not.

diuretics Drugs that help the body get rid of excess water and salt.

esophagitis An inflammation of the esophagus that may result from anticancer treatments.

esophagus The first part of the digestive tract linking the mouth to the stomach.

estrogen A female sex hormone.

gastrointestinal Having to do with the digestive tract, which includes the mouth, esophagus, stomach, and intestines.

gene The basic unit of inheritance in the cells.

germs   A general term used to describe all viruses, bacteria, and microscopic fungi.

hallucinations   A perception unaccompanied by reality, e.g., hearing voices when no one is present.

heparin   A substance that prevents blood coagulation.

Hodgkin's disease   A type of lymphoma, or cancer, that arises in the lymph nodes.

immune system   The bodily system that protects the body from infection by foreign substances. It includes the thymus, spleen, lymph nodes, bone marrow, and antibodies.

infusion   Slow and/or prolonged intravenous delivery of a drug or fluids.

intravenous (IV)   A tube that allows liquid to be dripped directly into the vein.

leukemia   Cancer found in the bone marrow.

lymphocytes   A type of white cell with a large, circular nucleus. When an infection occurs, lymphocytes multiply in the lymph nodes and attack the germs.

lymph system   Network that circulates fluid to bathe each cell; produces and stores cells that fight off germs and infections.

malignant tumor   A cancerous tumor.

menopause   A definite stoppage in menstruation; menopause usually occurs between the ages of forty-five and fifty-five. Symptoms include irregular menstrual cycles, fatigue, and hot flashes.

metastasis   Spread of cancer from original site to somewhere else in the body.

morphine   A drug used to decrease pain levels.

mucositis   An inflammation of the mouth that causes a burning sensation.

mutation   A sudden structural change within a gene or chromosome of an organism resulting in the creation of a new character or trait.

pathology   The study of disease; pathology labs are where diseased tissue and its causes are examined.

platelets   Special blood cells that help stop bleeding.

port   A small plastic or metal container surgically placed under the skin and attached to a central-venous catheter inside the body. Blood and fluids can enter or leave the body through the port through a special needle.

prostate   Muscular gland at the neck of the bladder surrounding the urethra in males.

proteins   A very complex class of molecules found in all human organs. There are hundreds of different proteins, all of which have very specific jobs. In the blood, hemoglobin, albumin, and antibodies are the best-known proteins.

protocol   The steps of a particular medical treatment or procedure, given in a particular sequence, which are written down.

radiation therapy   Cancer treatment with radiation (high-energy rays).

red blood cells   Cells that supply oxygen to tissues throughout the body.

remission   The partial or complete disappearance of signs and symptoms of disease.

risk factor   A condition that increases a person's chance of developing cancer.

scan   To examine (a body or body part) with a CAT scanner or similar scanning apparatus.

spinal tap   Also known as a lumbar puncture; a procedure that removes small amounts of the cerebral spinal fluid that bathes the brain and spinal cord.

stem cells   Cells found in the bone marrow; they have the ability to multiply, and they generate all of the cells found in the blood.

stomatitis   Sores on the lining of the mouth.

tumor   An abnormal growth of cells or tissues. Tumors may
  be benign (noncancerous) or malignant (cancerous).
white blood cells   The blood cells that fight infection.

Where to Go for Help

American Cancer Society

The American Cancer Society is a voluntary organization with a national office and local units all over the country. This organization supports research, conducts educational programs, and offers many services to patients and their families. The American Cancer Society also provides free booklets on colorectal cancer and on sexuality. To obtain booklets, or for information about services and activities in local areas, call the Society's toll-free number, (800) ACS-2345 (227-2345), or the number listed under American Cancer Society in the telephone book. Its Web site is http://www.cancer.org.

Cancer Care Inc.

A not-for-profit organization that provides professional counseling, support, education, and telephone services to cancer patients and their families. It can also put you in touch with other patients and families so you can get support from people who are going through similar experiences.
275 7th Avenue
New York, NY 10001
(212) 302-2400
(800) 813-HOPE (813-4673)

e-mail: info@cancercareinc.org
Web site: http://www.cancercareinc.org

Cancer Information Service

The Cancer Information Service, a program of the National Cancer Institute, is a nationwide telephone service for cancer patients and their families and friends, the public, and health care professionals. The staff can answer questions in English or Spanish and can send free National Cancer Institute booklets about cancer. They also know about local resources and services. One toll-free number, (800) 4-CANCER (422-6237), connects callers all over the country with the office that serves their area. Its Web site is http://cis.nci.nih.gov.

Candlelighters

The Candlelighters Childhood Cancer Foundation is an organization of parents whose children have or have had cancer. This foundation provides services such as a youth newsletter and a parent information service.

Candlelighters Childhood Cancer Foundation
3910 Warner Street
Kensington, MD 20895
(800) 366-CCCF (366-2223)
(301) 962-3521
Web site: http://www.candlelighters.org

Candlelighters Childhood Cancer Foundation Canada is the Canadian liaison and educational arm of the international network of over 200 support groups for families of children with cancer and the medical and psychosocial professionals who serve them.

Candlelighters Childhood Cancer Foundation Canada
55 Eglinton Avenue East, Suite 401

Toronto, ON M4P 1G8
(800) 363-1062
(416) 489-6440
Web site: http://www.candlelighters.ca

Make-a-Wish Foundation
This organization works with families of terminally ill children. It provides the financial assistance and arrangements
necessary to grant a child's special wish, such as meeting a
favorite role model.
3550 North Central Avenue, Suite 300
Phoenix, AZ 85012
(800) 722-WISH (722-9474)
(602) 279-9474
Web site: http://www.wish.org

WEB SITES
To learn more about cancer and cancer research:

cancerfacts.com
http://www.cancerfacts.com

cancerpage.com—Cancer Information and Community
http://www.cancerpage.com

cancersource.com
http://www.cancersource.com

oncology.com: Online Action Against Cancer
http://www.oncology.com

For Further Reading

Canfield, Jack, Mark Victor Hansen, and Kimberly Kirberger. *Chicken Soup for the Surviving Soul: 101 Stories of Courage and Inspiration from Those Who Have Survived Cancer.* Deerfield Beach, FL: Health Communications, 1996.

Canfield, Jack, Mark Victor Hansen, and Kimberly Kirberger. *Chicken Soup for the Teenage Soul: 101 Stories of Life, Love and Learning.* Deerfield Beach, FL: Health Communications, 1997.

Canfield, Jack, Mark Victor Hansen, and Kimberly Kirberger. *Chicken Soup for the Teenage Soul II: 101 More Stories of Life, Love and Learning.* Deerfield Beach, FL: Health Communications, 1998.

Dorfman, Elena. *The C-Word: Teenagers and Their Families Living with Cancer.* Troutdale, OR: NewSage Press, 1994.

Drum, David. *Making the Chemotherapy Decision.* Los Angeles: Lowell House, 1996.

Ferris, Jean. *Invincible Summer.* New York: Farrar, Strauss, and Giroux, 1994.

Kaufman, Miriam. *Easy for You to Say: Q&A for Teens Living with Chronic Illness or Disability.* Buffalo, NY: Key Porter Books, Ltd., 1995.

Kent, Deborah. *The Only Way Out.* New York: Scholastic Inc., 1997.

Mason, K. *We Interrupt This Life: Leukemia Through a Child's Eyes.* Phoenix, AZ: Make-a-Wish Foundation, 1994.

McKay, Judith, and Nancee Hirano. *The Chemotherapy and Radiation Therapy Survival Guide.* Oakland, CA: New Harbinger Publications, Inc., 1998.

Patenaude, Dr. Robert. *Surviving Leukemia: A Practical Guide.* Buffalo, NY: Key Porter Books, Ltd., 1999.

Potter, John F. *How to Improve Your Odds Against Cancer.* 2nd ed. Hollywood, FL: Lifetime Books, Inc., 1998.

Winawer, Sidney, and Moshe Shike. *Cancer Free: The Comprehensive Cancer Prevention Program.* New York: Simon & Shuster, 1995.

Index

L

leukemia, 58–60, 63, 70–71
  acute lymphoblastic (ALL),
    59–60, 63, 64, 65
  acute nonlymphoblastic
    (ANLL), 59–60
light, sensitivity to, 56
Lipton, Jeffrey, 85–88
liver, 6, 17, 56
lymph glands/nodes, 70–71, 84
lymphoma, 70–71

M

mammogram, 9, 83
meningitis, 57
menopause, premature, 35, 85
metastasis, 66
mouth, sores in, 31–33, 57, 61,
  64, 69, 73, 85
MRI (magnetic resonance
  imaging), 55, 57, 70
mucositis, 31–32
muscle tension and release, 45

N

nausea, 24–26, 55, 61, 64, 67,
  69, 71, 77, 83, 85
non-Hodgkin's lymphoma,
  70–71, 72
nurses, 2, 39, 69, 87

O

oncologist, 2, 4, 35, 55, 64, 68,
  69, 72, 73, 77, 79–89
  questions for, 18–20
outpatient, 18, 64, 76

P

paralysis, facial, 55, 57
PICC (peripherally inserted
  central-venous catheter),
  15, 69, 73
port, 16, 62, 64
pregnancy, 36–37
protocol (treatment plan), 14–15,
  18, 22, 37, 61, 62, 64,
  72, 76, 87–88
  ICE, 56, 57
psychologist, 2, 40

R

radiation, 8
  therapy, 18, 34, 56, 65,
    70, 74
rays, ultraviolet, 7
regression, 52–53, 82
relapse, 62, 65, 88
relaxation techniques, 44–50
remission, 61, 65, 71

S

scoliosis, 54–55, 57
seizures, 56–57
sexual activity, 35–37
siblings, 50–51
side effects
  emotional, 2–3, 40–53
  nervous system, 37
  physical, 2–3, 22–39, 50, 73
  preventing, 36, 85
skin and nails, dryness of, 33–35
sleep disturbance, 40–41, 50
smoking, 7, 8

Acknowledgments

Our thanks to all the patients, children, teens, and adults whom we interviewed for this book. Our thanks to their families as well. A special thank-you goes to Liz Nichols, Dr. Mark Greenberg, Dr. Ellen Warner, and Dr. Jeffrey Lipton.

About the Authors

Sandra and Owen Giddens make their home in Toronto, Canada. Owen is a doctor of psychology and Sandra is completing her doctorate in education. Owen has a private practice specializing in trauma and pain management. He is also a licensed marital, family, and child therapist. Sandra is a special education consultant for the Toronto District School Board.

DATE DUE

MAY 2 2 2002		
JUL 0 9 2002		
DEC 0 2 2003		
DEC 1 8 2003		

The Library Store   #47-0102